Oh! EYE SEE

Oh! EYE SEE

AN INSIGHT TO EYE CARE

Authored By,

Dr. Renuka Chavan

WINGS PUBLICATION INTERNATIONAL
WE GIVE WINGS TO YOUR DREAM!

Disclaimer

WINGS PUBLICATION INTERNATIONAL
WE GIVE WINGS TO YOUR DREAM!

Registered Office- 907-Sneh Nagar, Sapna Sangeeta Road,
Agrasen Square, Indore – 452001 (M.P.), India

Website: http://www.wingspublication.com

Email: mybook@wingspublication.com

First Published by WINGS PUBLICATION 2024

Title : Oh! Eye See

Price : Rs. 499 | $ 11.99

ISBN : 978-93-6006-574-4

Dedication

I dedicate my book to my beloved Late Grandfather
NANA- Shri. Haribhau Dnyandev Patil.

Thank you, my most respected Nana, for inculcating in me the habit of reading and nurturing books, right from my early childhood days. Thank you for always being there with me as my guardian angel.

Acknowledgements

There is a huge contribution of all the people in my life, in making me the empowered person I am today.

My Deities-

Shri Ganapati and Shri Datta Guru Maharaj.

Om Ganapataye Namah

Jai Gurudev Datta.

My Paternal Grandparents-

Late Shri Haribhau Patil and Late Shrimati Sushila Patil, I am grateful to them for being an ideal example themselves, of how to lead an ethical and honest life! I am thankful to them for imbibing in me the core beliefs of truth, self -respect, perseverance and kindness. I just wish, you both were here today to hold me and my book, but I know you are always watching over me forever.

My Maternal Grandparents-

Shrimati Shalini Patil and Late Shri Dhondiram Patil, I am grateful for your unconditional love, support and blessings.

Shri Shri Ravi Shankar Gurudev-

I am so thankful to you for enriching my life with the meditations and principles of Art of Living! Jai Gurudev!

My Parents-

Dr. Vivek Patil and Mrs Pratibha Patil, I am grateful to you for raising me well and imparting me with the best values.

My Parents in law-

Dr. Dilip Chavan and Mrs. Alka Chavan, I am grateful to you for your love, blessings and encouragement.

My Husband-

Dr. Niranjan Chavan, I am forever thankful to you for being besides me as my admiring comrade in all my endeavours.

My darling Son- Jotiraditya Chavan, I am so grateful to you for being my strongest champion. You inspire me to become better and achieve better than the before, always.

My respected Uncle and Aunty Dr. Shri P. D. Patil Sir, Chancellor of Dr.D.Y.Patil University, Pune and Dr. Mrs. Bhagyashree Patil Madam, Pro Chancellor Dr.D.Y.Patil University, Pune and Chairperson and Managing Director of Rise n' Shine Biotech - I am so grateful to you for the encouragement you have provided me in my formative years in the form of education and your magnificent larger than life persona! I always look up to you as my role models in how to fulfill all the dharmas of life in the most ideal way.

My Brother and Sister-in-law - Dr. Prithviraj Patil and Dr. Neha Patil;

I am grateful to you for being the sturdy pillars of unconditional love and support in my life.

My Brother-in-law and Sister-in-law - Dr. Jayant Choure and Dr. Arti Choure-

I am grateful to you for being an amazing example of how to live a fruitful life with academic excellence and morals.

All my school teachers of Modern English School Sangli, Maharashtra; college teachers of Willingdon College Sangli, Maharashtra; teachers of Chate coaching classes Sangli, Maharashtra; professors and lecturers of Dr.D.Y.Patil Medical College, Pune, Maharashtra and Lions NAB Eye Hospital Miraj, Sangli Maharashtra;

Seniors and colleagues of Jalgaon Ophthalmological Association, Jalgaon Maharashtra and my professional seniors and colleagues all over India-

I am grateful to you for the constant encouragement and the education you have given me throughout my life. You have added to my knowledge in the best possible way.

I am eternally grateful to my Coaches-

Dr. Meghana Dixit for the magnificent brain rewiring techniques.

Mrs Nayan Agrawal for the powerful processes.

Mrs Rashmi Sawant for the energetic breathing exercises.

Dr. Shilpa Bhansali for the calming meditations.

Mr. Jignesh Paddhiyar- For the superb life coaching, graphotherapy, encouragement for book writing, also suggesting the title!

Dr. Purva Deshpande- For making me aware of my potential and for being confident that one day I will be an author! You saw it in me when I could not.

All my friends and relatives, I am grateful to you for your incredible company and constant support. Thank you for looking at me like I am the super women who can literally achieve anything! You are the wind beneath my wings!

I am grateful to all my patients for your love and trust in me!

Dr. Kailash Pinjani, founder of Wings publication, I am grateful to you for your trust in this book and for being the receiver of the constant accountability provided by me, throughout my journey of book writing.

Ms Manika Singh, CEO of Wings Publication, Ms Varsha Mane, Ms Chinmayee Bhate, Dr. Deepak Parbat, Mr. Abhas Mangal and the entire team of Wings Publication for your expert professional guidance.

To all my supporting staff in my hospital and at my home, I am grateful to you for your timely and sincere services.

I am grateful to each and every person in my life for the progress and learnings in this lifetime.

Preface

I am very thankful to you my dearest reader for selecting this book! I have written this book with a pure intention of increasing your awareness about the eyecare. I assure you that after reading this book, you will be well versed with the eye care methods, so that you will be in a better position to care for yourself and your loved ones!

Our eyes are the gateway to the infinite universe. So, the health of our eyes is of prime importance.

“Beauty lies in the eyes of the beholder”- Plato.

Our perception of the environment is created primarily by what we see. It is a common saying- ‘The first impression is the last impression!’ and our eyes play a vital role in creation of the impression of whatever we come across throughout the day.

In my daily practice of Ophthalmology, I come across patients who suffered an eye discomfort or an injury, because they didn’t know in the first place that certain activities might harm their eyes. If they were already well acknowledged with the care taking of the eyes, the extent of discomfort or injury might have been reduced or totally avoided.

This realisation inspired me to write this book!

As a doctor, it's been my primary aim to serve the society through my work in the field of Ophthalmology.

An awareness created in the society will help many to take care of themselves. Spiritually 'awareness' is of utmost importance. It is said- awareness of self leads to awareness of God!

This book is my humble contribution at creating awareness for the betterment of the society.

As a kid, I was always mesmerised by the story books! As I grew up, books became an inevitable part of my being.

Books are a person's best friends.

Today, when I am presenting my book to the world, I am immensely happy and blessed as an author.

Ophthalmology is my passion and books are my first love! So, my book, 'Oh! Eye See', an insight to eye care is written with the utmost love and passion! As much as I have enjoyed writing this book, I am sure you too will enjoy reading it!

Testimonials

This is the ultimate guide to taking care of your eyes and making sure that they are healthy and well cared for. We also learn about various ailments regarding the eyes and how to prevent or treat them. An amazing effort by Dr. Renuka in writing this book for everyone's benefit.

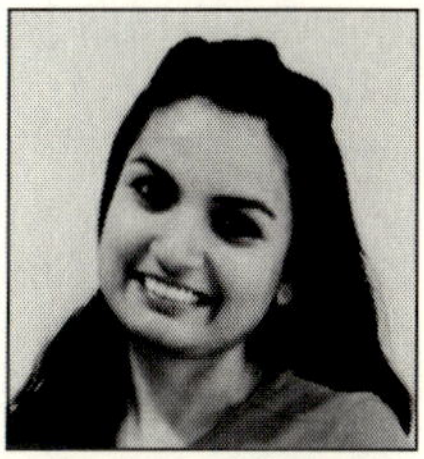

Manika Singh

Best Selling Author of "DECODING FITNESS" & "CHAKRA ENTREPRENEUR"

This book is a must on everyone's shelf. For an organ as delicate as the eyes, not a lot of people know how to care for them. With this book, care for eyes becomes an easy task and it's something everyone needs in their life. Care of eyes is an essential routine in everyone's life and this book will provide the correct guidance for it.

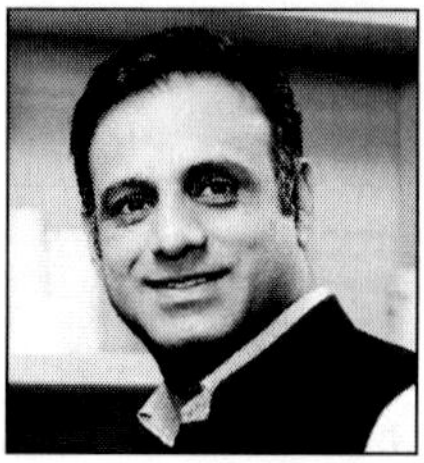

Dr. Kailash Pinjani

Best Selling author of "Decoding Fitness" & "CATCH THE SHARK"

Caring for the eyes is a necessary task. Everyone should be able to care for their eyes. This book not only gives an insight into how to care for eyes but also the different structures of eyes, of the history of eyes and ophthalmology. With this book, the health of eyes will be decoded and make it easy to maintain them.

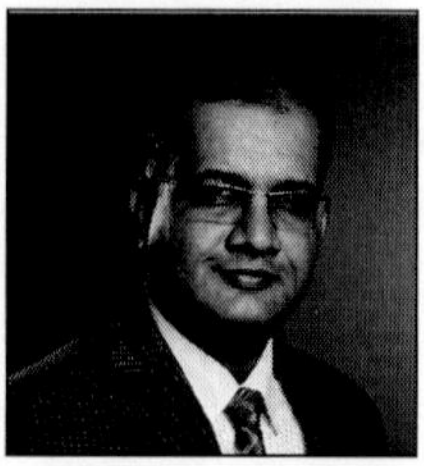

Dr. Deepak Parbat

Best Selling Author of "WELL DONE! YOU ARE HIRED" & "A MONK IN SUIT"

Index

CHAPTER 1

Let's know about our eyes

Eyes are the windows to our souls and the canvas to our emotions... Having inspired poets and lovers for centuries, eyes still hold the supreme position to enchant writers and philosophers. Being an Ophthalmologist, I am always privileged to be in the vicinity of these beautiful eyes and to observe their multiple facets!

History of the Ophthalmology:

The Ophthalmology branch of medicine is a very unique branch that is always at the forefront of embracing newer technology and inventions for the betterment of society. Let's have a look at its glorious evolutionary journey since the ages.

A] Prehistoric and Classical Era (3000 BC to AD 476) –

1) Ancient Egypt-

    The practice of Ophthalmology has been documented since ancient times. Its existence can be traced back to Ancient Babylon with the reference to the eyes made in the Code of Hammurabi (2250BC).

    However, it was not until Ancient Egypt that the first

known written record of medical treatment of eye diseases was discovered in the Ebers Papyrus, which dates back to 1550 BC.

The Eye of Horus, later known as Wedjat, became one of the most popular amulets worn by the Egyptians and featured as a prominent symbol of healing, protection and good health.

2) Ancient Greek

Pre- Hippocratic era-

Here, the anatomical conception of the eye was mainly speculative. Alcmaeon of Croton (540-500 BC), a prominent philosopher-physician at the time, was widely regarded as the first to examine and describe the human eye. He and others described the eye comprises of the two layers-

An outer layer consisting of the sclera and cornea.

An inner layer bordered anteriorly by the pupil with fluid at the centre.

3) Hippocratic era-

The Hippocratic Corpus, a collection of approximately 60 early Ancient Greek medical works by Hippocrates (460-375BC), further advanced the ideas of Alcmaeon of Croton.

The eye was now described as comprising three layers-

A thick outer layer

A thinner middle layer

An inner thinnest layer.

Aristotle (384- 322 BC) further put forth the existence of this anatomical framework based on animal dissections and described the optic nerve as a duct connecting the eye with the membranes of the brain.

4) Hellenistic (Post Hippocratic) era-

The invasion of the Achaemenid Empire in 330 BC by Alexander the Great ushered in the Hellenistic era in which Greek cultural influence and power reached its zenith. Herophilus (330-260BC), a Greek physician, showed special interest in the eye. His work was inherited and quoted by subsequent scholars such as Celsus, Rufus and Galen. Through their work, the existence of further ocular structures was given a clear recognition, including the lens, which was called a drop-like body named crystalloids and a large empty space, which was called locus vacuus containing 'humor', representing the anterior chamber of the eye.

5) Ancient India –

Sushruta, the most celebrated physician and surgeon in India, is widely regarded as the Father of Ophthalmology. Current consensus places him around the fifth century

BC (a century earlier than Hippocrates). He devoted a complete volume of his experiences on ocular anatomy and pathology to the final sections of Sushruta Samhita, a monumental treatise on surgery. This compilation, referred to as the Uttara Tantra, contained elaborate descriptions of 76 eye diseases such as glaucoma (Gambhirika), uveitis (Adhi-mantha), cataract (Kacha) and trichiasis (Pakshma-kopa). In addition, Sushruta described in the Samhita of what may be the first cataract extraction using a sharply curved needle used to loosen and push the cataract out of the field of vision.

6) Ancient Rome-

The Greco-Roman physicians made remarkable anatomical discoveries of the eye and refined the surgical instruments and techniques. Among these, Celsus (25BC to 50AD) was the first to systemically deal with ophthalmology, with related manuscripts preserved to the present day. Through his pioneering work, De Re Medica, Celsus earned the reputation as one of the greatest contributors to ophthalmology during the Roman empire. Certain views, such as the crystalline lens as the central organ of vision and cataract as an opaque concretion between the lens and the iris, were still held with high regard, and these persisted through the Middle Ages.

B] The Middle Ages (AD 476 to 1450)-

Arabian Era-

During this period, incomparably more manuscripts on Ophthalmology were written in Arabic compared to Latin, Greek and other European languages combined. Hunayn Ibn Ishaq Al-Ibadi (809-873) wrote the Book of the Ten Treatises of the Eye, which built upon the work of Greek scholars and delineated the first detailed anatomical illustration of the eye.

Revolutionary work in the field of optics was achieved by Ibn Al–Haytham (965-1040) through his book of optics known as Kitab al-Manazir. In it, he described the correct theory of vision in which the seeing process was facilitated by the light rays radiating from an object to the eye.

The previous practices of the Greco-Roman physicians were deemed crude and frowned upon by many of the leading figures in the medieval Arabist age. Guided by scientific methods, the flourishing science of Ophthalmology serves as the foundation of European science and has endured well into the Modern Era.

C] Early Modern Era (AD 1450 to 1800)-

The 14th century witnessed the beginning of the Renaissance, a fervent period of rebirth in science, culture and politics for Europe. The first physicians specialising in Ophthalmology were known as 'Oculists', a term adapted from the Latin word oculus, meaning eye.

Many great leaps in ocular anatomy were achieved.

Giacomo Berengario (1460-1530) accurately described the conjunctiva as a separate ocular structure for the first time.

Andreas Vesalius (1514-1564) discovered that the human crystalline lens, when removed, functioned as a convex lens.

The true anatomical position of the lens behind the pupil was later demonstrated by Hieronymus Fabricius ab Aquapendente (1533-1619) around 1600.

This concept gained support in the 18th century after being advocated by Antoine Maitre-Jan (1670-1725), who is widely regarded as the father of French Ophthalmology.

It was also around this time that the first full cataract extraction in the Western world was performed by Charles Saint Yves (1677-1731) in 1707.

Jacques Daviel (1696-1762) further refined this technique and contributed much to the dissemination of extracapsular cataract extraction.

George Bartisch (1535-1607), a German physician who wrote extensively on eye disease in the 16th century, was perhaps the most well-known oculist of his time and is considered to be the Father of Modern Ophthalmology. His comprehensive work featured 92 full-page woodcuts depicting eye disease, surgical methodology and instrumentation.

In 1722, Saint Yues published a treatise on eye pathologies that became an established pillar of the French School of Ophthalmology.

In the 18th century, Johann Gottfried Zinn (1727-1759), a German anatomist who is often referred to as the father of ocular anatomy, provided the first detailed, comprehensive layer-by-layer anatomy of various ocular structures.

In India, Maharaja Serfoji Raje Bhosale II (1777- 1832) contributed to the Ophthalmology. He was the ruler of Thanjavur from 1798 to 1832. He was a descendant of the Chhatrapati Shivaji Maharaj's half-brother Venkoji Raje, who founded the Thanjavur Maratha Dynasty in 1675. Serfoji Raje II was the 10th ruler of the Venkoji Raje.

He was a scholar, philosopher and humanist. He established Dhanvantari Mahal, a hospital that took care of the patients of all specialities. It was also a research institute which produced herbal medicines for humans and animals.

Serfoji Raje took special care to treat eye ailments. It is said that the king himself was an expert in treating eye diseases and performing cataract surgeries. Ophthalmic records of 44 patients were found in which various eye diseases were diagnosed, and treatment modality was explained.

D] Modern Era (1800 AD to present)-

The early 19th century saw the discipline of Ophthalmology

becoming a well-defined area of practice.

Austrian Ophthalmologist Georg Joseph Beer (1763-1821) in 1812 founded the first university department of Ophthalmology in the general hospital of Vienna and established the first medical school and clinic dedicated to the treatment of eye disease.

The first dedicated ophthalmic hospital was opened in London, England in 1805. Currently known as Moorfields Eye Hospital, it was initially founded as the London Dispensary for curing the diseases of the eye and the ear.

The mid-19th century saw the invention of the direct ophthalmoscope by Hermann von Helmholtz (1821-1894), a German physicist and physician, in 1851, which offered unprecedented diagnostic capabilities and revolutionised the practice of Ophthalmology.

Sir William Bowman (1816-1892) from Moorfields founded the Ophthalmological Society of the UK, now known as the Royal College of Ophthalmologists, in 1880 and provided a central organisation to learn through meetings and presentations.

Allvar Gullstrand (1862-1930), a Swedish Ophthalmologist, invented the slit lamp in 1911 with Carl Zeiss (1816-1888) of Germany using the Nernst electric bulb. This groundbreaking invention, which allowed a magnified, illuminated view of the interior of the eye with a slit of light, has acquired the greatest importance to the practical ophthalmologist.

Advancements in various branches of Ophthalmology accelerated during the 20th century.

The 20th century also ushered in a golden age for cataract surgery due to the contributions of the pioneers, most notably Sir Harold Ridley (1906- 2001) and Charles Kelmann (1930-2004).

Ridley performed the first intraocular lens implant in 1949. Nearly two decades later, Kelman introduced phacoemulsification in 1967.

The technology has since revolutionised the nature of cataract surgery and transformed it into a faster procedure, with a shorter postoperative recovery period and reduced duration of admission in the hospital.

THE STRUCTURE OF AN EYEBALL-

Knowing the structure of the eyeballs will help us to understand better how it works. Eyeballs are very fragile in their constitution yet very powerful in their functioning. When we know better about them, we will be in a better position to take care of them and protect them.

Eye anatomy

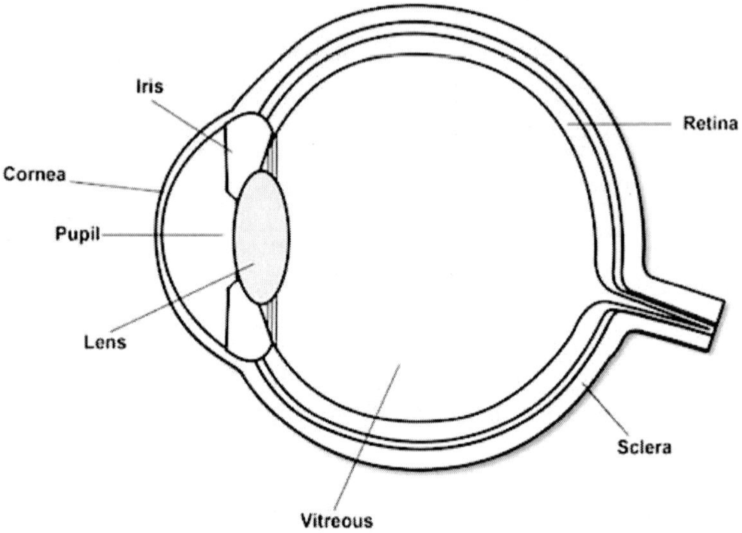

Eyeballs consists of the following structures-

A] ORBIT AND EYEBROWS-

Guess the answer to this riddle-

Two brothers are staying beside each other, but they cannot meet or see each other ever…

Answer- Yes, it's our eyes! They are in the bony cavities in the skull called orbits, which are separated in the centre by the nasal bridge! So our one eye can never see our another eye.

a) Orbits are the two cup-like cavities in the front of our skull in which eyeballs are situated. The skull provides a strong protection to the posterior side of the eyeballs.

Orbits also contain fat for the insulation and padding for the eyeballs, which work as shock absorbers in case of external pressure.

Orbits also host nerves, blood vessels, extraocular muscles and the lacrimal gland.

b) Eyebrows-

Hello, all you beautiful ladies with pretty arched eyebrows and all the handsome hunks with strong eyebrows!! Eyebrows are an important part of our looks. But there are also other important functions of eyebrows apart from giving you great looks!

The following are the functions of the eyebrows-

1) Role in facial configuration and ornamentation.

2) Role in facial expressions- various emotions are expressed by the movements of eyebrows.

   By elevating eyebrows- fright, pleasure and surprise are expressed.

   By depressing and drawing together of eyebrows-

   Deep thought, anger or puzzlement are expressed.

3) Protective function of the eyebrows-

   By position and curvature, they help shield the eyes from the bright sunlight directly coming from above.

   Protects eyes from the sweat running down from the forehead.

They are extremely sensitive to external touch, so they help in the protection of the eyes and upper face by generating an early warning.

They help in extreme upper gaze and forceful closure of the eyelids.

B] EYELIDS AND EYELASHES-

a) Eyelids-

They are the shutters which protect the eyes from injuries and excessive light.

They help the tear film to spread evenly over the surface of the eyes and keep them moist.

Like eyebrows, they contribute to facial expressions, giving an idea about wakefulness and attention.

b) Eyelashes-

Long, fluttery eyelashes are desired by every girl! They add to the beauty quotient.

They protect the eyes by preventing the entry of dust particles into the eyes.

At their base, they host the glands, which secrete the oily secretions, forming an important part of the tear film.

C] CONJUNCTIVA, LACRIMAL APPARATUS AND TEAR FILM-

a) Conjunctiva-

It is the translucent mucous membrane which lines the inside of the lids and front of the eyeballs.

It has many mucin-secreting glands, which help to lubricate the movement of lids over the eyes and keep the tear film stable.

b) Lacrimal apparatus-

The lacrimal apparatus consists of a group of structures involved in the formation of tears and their transport.

The vintage hero might have said- *"Pushpa, I hate tears...!"* But we must love them as tears keep our eyes moist and prevent our cornea from drying.

We notice tears only when they roll down the eyes, but they are continuously formed in our eyes to keep them hydrated.

The structures constituting the lacrimal apparatus are-

1) The Main Lacrimal Gland is situated towards the upper and outer side of the eyeball inside the orbit.
2) Accessory lacrimal glands are situated behind the lids.
3) Tears are formed and distributed evenly and regularly with the help of the movement and blinking of the eyelids.

4) They are drained into the lacrimal sac present in the lower and inner side of the orbit via lacrimal punctum and canaliculi.

5) From the lacrimal sac, they are carried into the nose via a duct.

c) Tear film-

The most important function of the tear film is to form a perfectly smooth surface on the cornea and keep it moist along with the outer surface of the eye.

Tear film serves as the lubricant for the surface of the eye and lids.

It transfers the oxygen from the ambient air to the cornea.

It prevents infections due to its anti-bacterial properties.

It washes away debris and noxious irritants from the surface of the eyes.

It provides the pathway for the fighter cells (white blood cells) in case of an injury.

Tear film has a perfect balance of mucin layer, aqueous layer and lipid layer.

D] SCLERA AND EXTRAOCULAR MUSCLES-

a) Sclera means the white portion of the eyes. It forms the opaque 5/6th part of the external fibrous tunic of the eyeball.

Its whole outer layer is covered by a translucent capsule and also by the conjunctiva in the outer exposed part.

b) Extraocular muscles-

Do you remember the *'nimbooda'* song with the famous rolling of the eyes? All thanks to the extraocular muscles of the eyes, that the eyes could be rolled by the actress in all directions!!

Extraocular muscles are a total of six in number in each eye, and they play a pivotal role in the complex mechanism of the movement of the eyeballs in an extremely coordinated way.

Loss of coordination in between the movement of the extraocular muscles of both eyes leads to squinting.

E] CORNEA-

Ye Kaali Kaali Aakhein...

The cornea is transparent watch glass like anterior 1/6th of the eyeball.

It is perceived as the black circle in the eyes (or blue, green, or brown, depending upon ethnicity or genetics) due to the colour of the iris behind it.

Its main function is to act as a pivotal refractive medium, to transmit light into the eyes so a clear image is formed. A complex mechanism is involved to keep the cornea clear.

The cornea also facilitates the transfer of medicines instilled in the eye to permeate inside the eye.

F) IRIS AND PUPIL-

a) Iris

It is a thin circular disc corresponding to the diaphragm of a camera.

It is the anterior part of a larger structure known as uveal tissue, which is predominantly concerned with the blood flow to the ocular tissues. Uveal tissue is the middle coat of the eyeball. It secretes a fluid known as aqueous humour and also maintains intraocular pressure.

b) Pupil

The central 3-4 mm opening in the iris is called the pupil. It regularises the amount of light reaching the retina.

Pupils are small at birth and largest during adolescence and tend to become smaller with increasing age.

Pupil tends to dilate during emotional stress and constricts during sleep. After death, they dilate completely.

G) LENS

The natural lens is a transparent crystalline disc-like structure present behind the iris. It is an important structure for clear vision and focusing on the objects.

The loss in its transparency is called a cataract, which usually develops any time after middle age, depending upon genetics and other factors.

Accommodation: It's the vital mechanism by which the lens can focus the near objects. It slowly gets weak after the age of 40.

H) VITREOUS HOMOR

a) Vitreous Homor

Our eye is a hollow structure. It's filled with a transparent jelly-like fluid in the centre, which also provides support to the eyeball.

I) RETINA AND OPTIC NERVE

a) Retina

It is a thin and the innermost layer of the eye.

It has special cells called photoreceptors. They are rods and cones.

They serve as sensory nerve endings for the visual stimuli. Adequate stimuli consist of the visible portion of the electromagnetic radiation spectrum, that is- The Light.

It lies in between ultraviolet and infrared portions from 400nm at the violet end to 750nm at the red end of the spectrum.

The white light consists of seven colours denoted by 'VIBGYOR' (violet, indigo, blue, green, yellow, orange, red).

Light falling on the retina is absorbed by the photosensitive pigments present in the rods and cones. This initiates photochemical changes, which trigger a sequence of events that initiate visual sensations.

Visual perceptions-

Visual perceptions are the functional elements of the vision- the sensations which result from stimulation of the retina and light.

They are of four types.

i) The light sense- It refers to the appreciation of light and all its gradations of intensity. Dark adaptation is the ability of eyes to adapt to the decreasing illumination. The rods are much more sensitive to low illumination than cones. Rods are used more in dim light, and cones are used more in bright light.

ii) The form sense- It is the ability to differentiate between the shapes of the objects. Cones play a major role in this faculty.

iii) Sense of contrast- It is the ability of an eye to perceive slight changes in the luminance between regions which are not separated by different borders.

iv) The Colour sense- It is the ability of an eye to discriminate between different colours excited by the light of different wavelengths. It is the function of cones and thus better appreciated in light. Cones perform this function with different types of pigments that absorb the primary colours- red, green, and blue.

b) Optic Nerve

Our eyes are like a camera that captures the images relayed to the brain through the optic nerves. The optic nerve, once damaged, never regenerates, so the diseases of the brain or the nerve itself involving atrophy of the nerve bring permanent blindness to the eyes.

CHAPTER 2

Nutrition and health of the eyes

Health is wealth! This holds true for our beautiful sparkling eyes, too! A healthy lifestyle can significantly reduce the risk of eye health problems. Foods that are high in antioxidants and vitamins play a key role in the health of our eyes.

A] Fruits-

1) Vitamin C-rich fruits-

Fruits like oranges, lemons, and grapefruit are rich in vitamin C. Vitamin C is vital in maintaining the body's form and connective tissue. The connective tissue known as collagen, found in the cornea of the eye, also needs vitamin C. Vitamin C also supports the health of blood vessels in the eye. It helps in combating age-related vision problems like macular degeneration and cataracts.

2) Berries-

Strawberries, cranberries, blackberries, and blueberries are great superfoods for the healthy functioning of the eyes. In berries, there are ample vitamins and minerals for maintaining eye health. Antioxidants called anthocyanins present in the berries also help prevent dryness, vision problems and age-related macular degeneration.

3) Bananas-

Bananas are one of the richest sources of potassium. Potassium is great for eye health and in preventing dryness, as it is an important component of the tear film and helps maintain film thickness.

Bananas are also a source of vitamin A, which is important for eye health as it protects the cornea.

4) Mango and Papaya-

Yellow yellow, great fellow!

Our king of fruits, mango, along with his friend papaya, are full of nutrients that help support healthy eyes. Vital nutrients in them are the antioxidants lutein and zeaxanthin. These act as a natural sunblock and absorb the excess light coming into the retina. They also protect the eyes from harmful blue light.

5) Apricots-

Apricots play a crucial role in ocular health as they contain vitamin A, vitamin C, vitamin E and beta-carotene. This is important for the night vision. They also help to absorb damaging blue light and ultraviolet light in order to protect the retina.

B] VEGETABLES

1)Carrots

Bunnies love carrots! But for the love of our pretty eyes, we should also turn into bunnies and consume carrots on a regular basis. They are commonly known to be good for eye health. They are rich in vitamin A and beta-carotene, which help in the well-being of the surface of the eyes and can also prevent eye infections.

2) Sweet Potatoes

Sweet potatoes are good sources of beta-carotene, potassium and fibre. The body converts beta-carotene to vitamin A, a nutrient that prevents dryness of eyes and night blindness and maintains healthy vision. They may even slow down the process of age-related macular degeneration.

3) Bell peppers

Bell peppers are a natural powerhouse that could help reduce the risk of age-related macular degeneration. They are rich, especially in vitamin C and carotenoids. Research suggests that the more carotenoids one eats, the greater protection from eye diseases.

4) Avocados

Avocados are the storehouse of vitamins and minerals. It is a superfood rich in antioxidants. Not only are they a great source of vitamins A, B6, C, E, and K, but they are also rich in lutein and zeaxanthin. Daily consumption is good for eye health and may delay the onset of age-related eye diseases.

5) Green leafy vegetables

Spinach and broccoli are leafy vegetables rich in both lutein and zeaxanthin. They are also rich in the eye-friendly vitamin C. The human body cannot make lutein and zeaxanthin, so they must be consumed in dietary sources.

C] Non-vegetarian sources

1) Fish

Salmon, tuna, sardines, halibut and trout are rich in omega-3 fatty acids.

Salmon is packed with essential fatty acids like DHA (docosahexaenoic acid).

DHA helps support retinal health, protecting it against dry eyes and macular degeneration.

2) Eggs

Eggs are an excellent source of zinc, an essential mineral for maintaining eye health. Zinc helps transport vitamin A from the liver to the retina, where it's converted to visual pigment rhodopsin that aids low-light vision. Eggs are also rich in lutein and zeaxanthin.

3) Oysters and Chicken

They are rich in zinc and vitamin A.

D] Exercises to promote eye strength

We know that exercising is good for the body's muscles. What about the exercises for the eye muscles? While there are no exercises to remove the spectacles, eye exercises can help with optimising visual skills.

While being under the doctor's care can provide more guidance on how to do the eye exercises, there are some exercises which can be done at home. While the improvement in the quantity of vision is not expected, with diligence, they can gradually help with focusing issues and eyestrain.

1) *Palming*- Palming is a yogic exercise that suggests relaxing the muscles around the eyes, reducing eye fatigue.

2) *Blinking*- When we spend time on digital devices, our blink rate goes down. Blinking pumps the oil glands in the eyelids, stimulating their lubricating secretions. It also helps spread the tears over the eyes.

   A blinking exercise involves closing the eyes, pausing for two seconds, and then opening them again. While the eyes are closed, the eyelids can be consciously squeezed tight for extra stimulation of oil glands.

3) *Pencil push-ups*- Pencil push-ups are commonly used to train the eyes to move in towards one another or converge while looking at near objects.

   To do a pencil push-up, hold a pencil at arm's length while wearing your best near-vision correction. Focus on the tip of the pencil. Slowly move the pencil towards your nose, keeping the tip of the pencil focused. Once a double image starts forming, draw it away from the eyes again. Repeat this slowly for five minutes twice a day.

4) *Near and far focus*- Alternating between near and far focus helps to train your focusing system to engage and relax appropriately.

   Hold your thumb 10 inches from your face and focus on it for 15 seconds. Alternatively, you can hold near objects with a letter on them to better engage your focusing system. After 15 seconds, shift your gaze to the target 20 feet (6 meters) away and hold your focus for 15 seconds again. Return to your thumb. Repeat for 5 minutes twice a day.

5) *Figure eight*- Tracking an object with the eyes can be challenging for some. To work on this, one can practice doing figure eight.

   Pick a point on the floor 10 feet away from you. With your eyes, trace an imaginary figure of eight. Continue for 30 seconds, and then switch directions.

CHAPTER 3

Screen usage and the eye strain

With the advent of the 21st century, there has been a revolution in the usage of digital devices and different types of screens.

The information technology sector has also flourished, leading to extensive use of computer screens throughout the day.

The last decade and a half has witnessed a faster evolution in the advance of mobile phones. All sections of society are heavily dependent on their mobile phone for the completion of their daily routines!

These lifestyle modifications have led to the emergence of a new lifestyle disease known as Computer vision syndrome.

Computer vision syndrome is a term used to describe a variety of vision-related symptoms that may be aggravated by the regular use of a computer for more than two hours a day.

The longer use of computers leads to a decrease in the blink rate.

This means that while working using a computer, we don't blink as often as we should.

Normal blink rate- 15 to 20 per minute.

During computer use, the blink rate decreases to 5-7 per minute.

Blinking is critically important for spreading tears to form an even film on the eye surface and also in refreshing this tear film.

Thus, in the absence of adequate blinking, eyes become dry and irritated.

Following is the mechanism of the reasons why the screens are the responsible element-

When we look at a distant object, our eyes are relatively relaxed and at rest.

But when we look at the computer screen continuously, our eyes get strained. Because-

Characters (pixels) on the computer screen do not have well-defined edges. They are brightest at the centre and diminish in intensity towards the edges.

This makes it very difficult for the eyes to focus.

Extensive focusing does not give much opportunity for the eye muscles to move, and this leads to eye strain, burning, and a feeling of tiredness in the eyes.

Causes of Computer Vision Syndrome-

1) Poor position in relation to computers.
2) Glare or reflection, fuzzy images that are too dim or too bright.

3) Use of glasses that are inappropriate for the user's position and distance from the screen.

4) Minor visual defects, such as astigmatism, that might go unnoticed, can be exaggerated with intense computer use.

5) Constant gazing at a near distance at the monitor leads to convergence fatigue.

6) Fixed posture while working for long hours.

7) Uncorrected visual defects.

8) Glare from lighting in the workplace and direct light coming inside from the exterior.

Symptoms of the Computer Vision Syndrome-

1) Double vision-

The patients typically complain of double vision due to tiredness of the eyes caused by a constant focus on the intermediate distance. There is a complex mechanism involved in which our eyes always work together to focus on objects similarly. So even if the eyes are two, we don't see two different images; we see only one image.

But in computer vision syndrome, the eyes are so tired that they refuse to work together, and thus, two different images can be seen for a few seconds or a few minutes.

2) Temporary near-sightedness-

Due to continuously focusing on the near distance, the

eyes take some time to focus on distant objects. When the focus is changed from prolonged near vision to suddenly at a distance, the intrinsic muscles of the eyes take time to focus. That is why intermittent breaks are recommended while working on the screen.

3) Dry eye-

When we look at a bright (or beautiful!!) object, we subconsciously start staring as our undivided attention goes to that bright or beautiful object. This action happens automatically. Here, the blinking is reduced for a few seconds or minutes.

But this action hampers the health of our eyes when we look at the illuminated screen for hours together every day.

The blinking action, which is necessary for the spread of tear film, gets reduced. Due to this, the eyes get dry, giving the symptoms of burning and grittiness in the eyes.

4) Decreased tolerance to the light.

Patients come with the classic complaints of being unable to tolerate even normal sunlight or household lights. In the computer professionals, who work on the screen for more than whooping 10 to 12 hours, due to regular gazing at the illuminated screen the eyes are always exposed to the bright light and don't get the break from intense lighting system to the comparatively soothing lighting environment. So, when they get exposed to even moderate sunlight or indoor lights, they experience photophobia.

5) Eye strain.

When our eyes look at a distant object, they are relaxed. Also, it's a natural gaze for them because, since the evolution of human beings till the last century, mankind has never worked extensively at a near distance, which is predominantly screen usage. Previously, we as humans were only hunters, gatherers, farmers, soldiers and likewise occupations involving more outdoor activities and focusing on distant objects. That is why even if our lifestyle has changed from outdoors to indoors and from focusing more on distance to focusing more on the near, our eyes are still the same as far as evolution is concerned. So focusing on the near and intermediate for a longer duration takes more effort and causes tiredness of the eyes or eyestrain.

6) Redness and watering from the eyes

The surface of our eyes is naturally well lubricated by the tear film. The ocular surface structures like conjunctiva and cornea are very sensitive and delicate. If proper moisture and hydration are not maintained, they suffer.

In computer vision syndrome, the blink rate is decreased, leading to the reduction in the spread of normal tear film. This causes redness and irritation in the eyes, which in turn causes the watering of the eyes. Also, due to the dryness of the eyes, a message is sent to the brain by the ocular nerves to produce excess tears to keep the eyes wet. So, the reflex tear production also occurs, causing even more watering.

7) Neck and Backaches.

Prolonged working in a fixed place with a table and chair is an essential part of a computer user's routine. If the height of the table or chair is faulty or the user is not sitting with the spine erect, it may cause postural pain in the neck and back.

Ideally, the computer user should use a proper chair to support the back. The elbows and wrists should be resting on the surface and should not be kept unsupported and hanging in the air. The neck should be in the shoulder line and not bending forward. The back should be touched to the chair and not bent forward. Taking a brisk walk for a few minutes in between the working hours will relieve the strained body muscles.

Prevention of Computer Vision Syndrome

1) Anyone who suspects the eye strain should have a thorough eye examination by an Ophthalmologist. As the severity of the dry eye is more severe in computer users than others, routine over-the-counter medications will not provide sufficient relief. The medications for the eyes should be

used only after examination by the ophthalmologist.

2) Blink more often- Computer users should make a conscious effort to blink more often.

   They should follow the rule of 20:20:20

   Every 20 minutes, look at a distance of 20 feet for 20 seconds.

   In practical life, for every 20 min, look outside the window at a distant object and slowly count to 20.

   This smaller lifestyle modification will take care of the maximum symptoms of computer vision syndrome.

3) Adjust the height of the desk or chair so that the middle of the computer screen is about 20 degrees below eye level, so the gaze is downwards. The screens placed on a higher surface cause an upward gaze and more exposure of the ocular surface, contributing to the dryness of the eyes.

4) Reduce glare- Direct the overhead lights away from the screen. Position your monitor so that all the windows are to the side rather than to the back or the front. Adjust the window blinds so that the sunlight is away from the screen and your eyes.

5) Avoid air drafts- Avoid sitting in front of an air conditioner facing its aircraft while working on the computer. The air coming out from the air conditioners is dry and lacks moisture, which is why people sitting in the AC rooms for

prolonged duration are susceptible to dry eyes. So, at least the dryness can be minimised by not facing the AC vents.

6) Take a break- Computer users can reduce fatigue by taking breaks from work and can benefit from taking a five-minute break for every 30 minutes of work.

Dryness of eyes due to screen usage-

When working on a computer or mobile for a longer duration, the following eye symptoms may occur-

1) Feeling of dryness, grittiness, burning and itching.
2) Sensitivity to light
3) Blurred vision
4) Excessive tear flow (caused by an imbalance in tear film).

This usually happens because of a deficiency in the watery component of the tear film, an increase in the tear film evaporation, or a combination of both of these.

Steps to manage dry eye in the screen users:

1) Check your medications- Talk to your doctor to see if prescription drugs might be causing dry eyes.
2) Nutrition- Eat three healthy meals and snacks every day.
3) Avoid pollution and irritants- Avoid rubbing the eyes, which disturbs the tear film and transfers irritants to your eyes.

4) Balance your hormones- Try eating more whole grains, less sugar and fewer processed foods. This will help to control insulin levels and keep inflammation under control.

5) Take special care with contact lenses-

   Keep contact lenses clean, and try not to wear them all the time.

6) Use artificial tears to provide more moisture and lubrication for the surface of the eyes.

7) Hydrate and humidify- If you are dehydrated, the fluid in your eyes can be depleted, so drink lots of fluids.

8) Blink- Try to blink consciously every five seconds, especially when staring at your computer screen or digital device.

CHAPTER 4

Eyes and hygiene

Our eyes are an important part of our health, but when it comes to hygiene, we often overlook proper care. A few healthy habits and additions to our daily routine can help us avoid contamination, infections and eye diseases.

The annual eye checkup is a very important part of taking care of the eyes. Most eye diseases, if caught early, are very much treatable, which is why it is so important to get yearly eye check-ups. Also, know your family history so that you can give yourself the chance to identify, monitor and treat any eye disease as early as possible.

a) Get an annual eye vision check-up-

Even if you have perfect vision, it is important to get your eye examined by an Ophthalmologist every year. They can see what you cannot see in your eyes.

Come prepared with your family history, as many eye diseases run in the families.

b) Remove your eye makeup each night before sleeping-

Excess debris from makeup can cause eye irritation and

redness. Use warm compresses, makeup removal wipes or natural alternatives such as coconut oil to remove makeup. To reduce puffiness, try finishing with a cool compress. Be sure to throw out expired or old makeup to reduce the risk of infection or irritation.

c) Wash your hands-

Common eye infections like conjunctivitis can be avoided with proper hand washing. Avoid sharing towels, makeup or medicated eye drops to prevent spreading bacteria to other people.

d) Quit smoking-

We all know that one of the best ways to improve health is to quit smoking. Smoking contributes to macular degeneration and cataracts.

Smoking can also cause dry eye when your tears are of poor quality and cause fuzzy vision, like a dusty windshield. In fact, people who smoke are twice as likely to develop age-related macular degeneration and two to three times more likely to develop cataracts than people who do not smoke.

e) Consume the carrots-

Carrots, spinach, apricots, sweet potatoes and fish contain nutrients that support a better vision.

These nutrients include-

Vitamin C

Vitamin E

Omega 3 fatty acids

Calcium

Zinc

Lutein and zeaxanthin are found in dark green leafy vegetables.

f) <u>Treat your contact lenses well-</u>

Always wash your hands with soap and water before removing your contact lenses. Use fresh solution every night. If you have been using the same storage case since you started wearing contact lenses, throw it out and replace it every three months. Do not use tap water to wash your contact lenses. It is not sterile and has microorganisms that can lead to serious infections. It is mandatory to remove the contact lenses before going to sleep.

Dispose of your contact lenses as recommended by your ophthalmologist. Do not try to extend the life of your contact lenses beyond the approved replacement schedule. Even though the lenses might feel ok in your eyes, the mucus starts building up on your contact lenses. This increases the risk of infection and inflammation. It may even result in corneal scarring and vision loss.

g) <u>Wear sunglasses-</u>

Sunglasses are a great style statement. But the main function is to protect the eyes from ultraviolet A (UVA) and ultraviolet B (UVB) rays, which in the long run can cause age-related macular degeneration and cataracts. So, your sunglasses should offer protection against UVA and UVB rays.

h) Keep the blood sugar levels controlled-

Diabetic retinopathy is a leading cause of vision loss and preventable blindness. Uncontrolled blood sugar levels are a risk factor. Yearly dilated retinal evaluation is necessary for diabetic patients.

i) Cleaning of hands before instilling the eyedrops and how to instil the eyedrops-

Eyedrops are the preferred mode of transmission of medicines for eye diseases. If hands are not washed before instilling eyedrops, it might lead to an infection in the eyes. Therefore, proper cleaning of the hands with a disinfectant soap is necessary.

To instil an eyedrop, first wash your hands. Instruct the patient to look up. Pull the lower eyelid down and then instill one drop inside the eyelid upon the lower side of the eye.

The eyes should be closed for a minute after that by the patient. Only one drop from the bottle of eyedrop should be put in as the eye only has a space of one drop in it. The second drop put in the eye always rolls outside the eye, causing wastage of the medicine.

If two or more eye drops are prescribed by an Ophthalmologist then a gap of five minutes should be given in between the two or three eyedrops.

j) Care and cleanliness of eyes in the postoperative patients of eye surgery.

1) The prescribed eyedrops should be administered inside the lower lid after thoroughly washing the hands. Never pull the upper lid to put the drops.

2) The eyedrops should be instilled at the exact time advised by the ophthalmologist.

3) Never rub the eyes and protect them from any trauma.

4) For two weeks after the surgery, clean the operated eye and face with antibiotic eye-cleaning wipes. Don't wash your face.

5) Dark protective goggles should be worn for two weeks after the eye surgery to protect the eyes from dust, sunlight, and trauma.

CHAPTER 5

Eyecare in children

Children are delicate compared to the adults and so are their eyes. So special care is required in children depending upon their age groups.

The immunity in children is also lesser compared to adults, which is why they might catch infections easily.

So here are some important points which the parents should take note of according to the age groups of children-

a) **Babies-**

Smoking can cause visual problems even in an unborn child's eyes.

Smoking is associated with a higher rate of bacterial meningitis, which in turn can cause severe vision loss. So active and passive smoking should be avoided by the pregnant ladies.

1) After birth-

For the first few months, the central vision is still developing. A newborn baby can see, but the connection between the brain and the retina is still developing. As the vision starts developing, they start seeing the objects in front of them.

2) Within three months of age-

In the first two months, the eyes of newborn babies might appear to have squint; this is usually normal as the eyes are not co-ordinated yet. As the visual coordination improves, the baby's eyes will work together to focus and follow objects. If you do not notice this happening consistently by the age of 3 months, talk to your Ophthalmologist.

3) Till the age of 5 months-

Till 5 months of age, babies are able to see how far the object is there from them as they are able to see better. They start developing depth perception. They may even remember the object.

4) Around 9 months-

At around 9 months of age, babies have developed their permanent eye colour. Eye colour depends on the amount and distribution of a brown pigment called melanin in the iris.

Light-coloured eyes at birth may darken if melanin develops in the eyes. Slight changes in eye colour are expected during the first 3 years of life.

b) Toddlers-

Observe if there is any misalignment in both eyes, which means if one eye looks straight ahead while the other looks inwards, outwards, upward or downwards. This might be a sign of squint. This can also be caught during the preschool vision examination by the Ophthalmologist.

It is important to vaccinate children against measles as the measles virus can harm the eyes.

Keep toddlers away from the chemicals and cleaning agents, as young children are more likely to get chemical burns. These burns are extremely dangerous as they cause permanent damage to the external as well as internal structures of the eyes. If there is a chemical injury in the children, wash the eyes with copious fluids and go to the nearest Ophthalmologist immediately.

c) School-age children-

There is farsightedness in many school children. In most cases, they do not need glasses. Children are usually able to focus on near as well as far using these intrinsic eye muscles. As the children grow, the length of the eyes increases, and the far-sightedness improves on its own. But more farsightedness can lead to strabismus and lazy eye if left uncorrected.

Delayed screen time causes myopia (near-sightedness) and straining of the eyes. It is seen in studies that near-sightedness is connected with near-work activities, including screen time.

Following are the signs of vision problems in childhood-

Loss of interest in the activities requiring sharp vision.

While reading, they lose track of the lines.

Turning the head to look at the front objects.

If one or more such signs are seen, consult an Ophthalmologist.

Poor vision, focusing problems, and jerky eye movements do not cause learning disabilities. They are caused by how the brain processes the information perceived via the eyes.

Children also get cataracts. It might be at birth or after birth. If proper treatment is not taken, abnormal connections are formed between the eyes and the brain that may become irreversible. The positive side is that cataracts in babies are discovered during eye screenings at birth or subsequent vision screenings by paediatricians.

Screen time should be limited as the blue light interferes with the sleep cycle, and a disturbed sleep cycle causes learning problems.

Colour blindness is more common in boys. It can be noticed when children fail to differentiate between different shades of the same colour.

d) <u>Teenagers and young adults-</u>

In children, trauma while playing is the most common cause of blindness. Cricket ball, football, and shuttle badminton are the common culprits.

More than 90 per cent of eye injuries can be prevented by protective goggles.

Children should wear sports eye protectors made with polycarbonate lenses for baseball, basketball, football, tennis, badminton, paintball and other activities with the risk of an injury.

Contact lenses should be avoided by teenagers as they cannot take proper care of them. This puts them at a higher risk of getting infections. If teenagers are using contact lenses, the proper care should be monitored by the parents.

Good vision is imperative for the child's overall academic and physical growth. Regular eye check-ups are quintessential for school-going kids!

CHAPTER 6

Common eye ailments

In this chapter, I am going to give you an overview of common eye diseases and what care should be taken if such diseases occur.

A] **Infective Conjucntivitis:**

Gulabi aankhein jo teri dekhi, sharabi ye dil ho gaya..!

Conjunctivitis, commonly known as pink eye, is the infection and inflammation of the conjunctiva, which is a transparent mucous membrane covering the anterior surface of the eyeball and the posterior surface of the eyelids.

The infection can be due to-

1) Bacteria

2) Virus

3) Fungus

4) Parasite

5) Chlamydia

Among the above types, bacterial and viral conjunctivitis are the most common.

Conjunctivitis is a communicable disease that spreads by contact with infective material coming out of the infected person's eyes.

It does not spread by looking into the eyes of the infected person, which is a very common myth.

Symptoms-

1) Redness

2) Watering

3) Sticky discharge

4) Gritty sensation

5) Swelling of eyelids

Care and prevention

1) The patient is isolated in a room for 3 to 5 days to avoid contact with other family members. Patients should rest in this phase and should not spend time on the screen as it leads to more irritation of the eyes.

2) Frequent hand washing by the patient and other family members.

3) Wash the clothes of the patient separately.

4) Use of goggles to minimise touching of the eyes by the patient of his own eyes which might transfer the infective

material in the house.

5) Regularly instilling eyedrops and taking medication prescribed by an Ophthalmologist. In the epidemic of conjunctivitis, many patients self-treat themselves by purchasing the medications without an examination from the Ophthalmologist. This might lead to the usage of unindicated eye drops and medications, leading to an increase in the severity and recovery time.

B] Cataract: Commonly known as motiya-bindu.

Cataract is a very common age-related eye disease caused by opacification of the crystalline lens in the eye.

Risk factors:

1) Increasing age
2) Sunlight (especially the UVA and UVB components)
3) Severe diarrhoeal dehydration
4) Vitamin A, C, and E deficiency
5) Diabetes
6) Smoking
7) Corticosteroid intake
8) Genetic
9) Eye trauma

10) In children- paediatric cataracts due to genetic and developmental health problems.

Symptoms-

1) Blurring of vision
2) In the late phase, white opacity is in the centre.
3) Doubling of the vision by the affected eye.
4) Frequent changes in the spectacle number and vision do not improve completely, even with the change in the spectacles in the later stages.
5) Coloured halos
6) Decrease in the contrast sensitivity.

Complications

If left untreated, cataracts become mature, and the hyper-mature leads to complete loss of vision, inflammation of the eyes, and an increase in the pressure of the eyes, causing optic nerve damage, leading to permanent loss of vision.

Treatment-

Surgery is the only treatment for cataracts. In cataract surgery, the cataract is removed, and the intraocular lens is implanted inside the eye. This lens is very different from the contact lens and is not removable. The intraocular lens is implanted inside the eyes, whereas the contact lens is on the surface of the cornea.

Phacoemulsification (commonly known as phaco) is the most common and recent technique of cataract surgery.

Cataract surgery is a planned and daycare surgery. Patients should plan it in time before the cataract matures, leading to an emergency.

The newer types of intraocular lenses offer better visual rehabilitation post-cataract surgery. Spectacle usage minimises after the surgery.

Care after cataract surgery-

Care and cleanliness of eyes in the postoperative patients of eye surgery.

- The prescribed eyedrops should be administered inside the lower lid after thoroughly washing the hands. Never pull the upper lid to put the drops.
- The eyedrops should be instilled at the exact time advised by the ophthalmologist.
- Never rub the eyes and protect them from any trauma.
- For two weeks after the surgery, clean the operated eye and face with antibiotic eye-cleaning wipes. Don't wash your face.
- Dark protective goggles should be worn for two weeks

after the eye surgery to protect the eyes from dust, sunlight, and trauma.

C] <u>Glaucoma</u>

It is commonly known as kala motiya in Hindi or kaach-bindu in Marathi.

Glaucoma, by definition, is a chronic progressive optic neuropathy caused by a group of ocular conditions which lead to damage to the optic nerve with loss of visual function.

The common risk factor is raised intraocular pressure. A sustained increase in the intraocular pressure is due to the increased production of aqueous humour or difficulty in its exit.

Symptoms:

1) Pain in the eyes, its severity depending upon the type of glaucoma.
2) Haloes are seen around the sources of light.
3) Loss of vision prominently in the peripheral region.
4) Nausea or vomiting in the sudden increase of intraocular pressure.
5) Redness and tiredness in the eyes for a long time
6) Sudden and severe headache.

People of any age group can get glaucoma. However, people

beyond the age of 40 years are more prone. There are no signs or symptoms in the early stage, but it can be easily diagnosed during a regular, non-invasive eye examination. Early diagnosis of glaucoma has a better chance of visual prognosis.

Treatment generally includes anti-glaucoma eyedrops, and surgery is seldom required in the cases uncontrolled on the anti-glaucoma medication.

D] Diabetic and hypertensive retinopathy-

Diabetes and hypertension are very common these days in the population due to lifestyle changes. They pose a serious and threatening effect on the various organs of the body.

In the eyes, these diseases affect the retina the most. They affect the small vessels in the retina causing swelling and bleeding in the retina, leading to the diminision of the vision or permanent vision loss.

Symptoms-

1) Decreased vision.
2) Frequent changes in the spectacle number.
3) Floating spots or dark strings in the vision line.
4) Dark areas in the vision
5) Loss of vision.

Prevention and care

Diabetic and hypertensive retinopathy can be picked up on the regular eye examinations. Controlled blood sugar levels and blood pressure also contribute to better retinal care.

Treatment includes the consumption of antioxidants and multivitamins to improve the retinal health.

In advanced cases, intravitreal injections, retinal lasers and retinal surgery are done depending on the severity.

E] <u>Dry eyes.</u>

Dry eyes are a common condition that occurs when the tears are not able to provide enough lubrication for the eyes.

Tears can be inadequate and unstable for many reasons. For example, if enough tears are not produced or if poor quality tears are produced. Inflammation and damage to the eye surface are caused by lesser quantity tears or poor-quality tears.

Having dry eyes is very uncomfortable. There is stinging, burning and irritation of the eyes. Dry eyes are commonly experienced by people sitting In an air-conditioned room for long hours, as the air from the air conditioners is dry. It is also seen in people using screens for long hours as the blink rate decreases and the tear film is inadequately formed.

Symptoms

1) Burning, stinging, scratchy sensation in the eyes

2) Sensitivity to the light
3) Redness in the eyes
4) Dust particle-like sensation in the eyes
5) Difficulty in wearing contact lenses
6) Difficulty in driving at night
7) Blurred vision
8) Eye fatigue

Causes

Dry eyes are caused by many things that disrupt the healthy tear film.

There are three layers in the tear film

Oily layer

Watery layer

Mucus layer.

This combination is responsible for a smooth and uniform layer of tears on the surface of the eyes.

Reasons for the tear film dysfunction are many, including hormonal changes, autoimmune disorders, eyelid glands not functioning properly and allergic disorders.

Decreased tear film production and increased tear film evaporation are also responsible for dry eyes in some people.

Tear glands and tear ducts-

The tear glands, called the lacrimal glands, are located above each eyeball and continuously supply the tear fluid that's spread across the surface of the eyes each time we blink. Excess fluid drained into the nose through tear ducts.

Decreased tear production by the glands-

Dry eyes occur when enough tears are not produced. Common causes include-

1) Ageing
2) Certain medical conditions include Sjogren's syndrome, allergic eye disease, rheumatoid arthritis, lupus, scleroderma, sarcoidosis, thyroid disorders and vitamin A deficiency.
3) Certain medicines include anti-histaminics, decongestants, hormonal replacement therapy, and antidepressants.
4) Also, in the people taking medication for high blood pressure, acne, birth control and Parkinson's disease.
5) Corneal nerve desensitivity is caused by contact lens use and nerve damage.

Increase tear evaporation:

The oily secretions produced by the meibomian glands of the eyelids are responsible for the stability of the tear film. The clogged meibomian glands are responsible for the increased evaporation.

Common causes of evaporative dry eye diseases include-

1) Meibomian gland dysfunction.
2) Decreased blink rate caused in the Parkinsonism, concentrating overtly during certain activities, driving or looking at the computer or mobile screen.
3) Eyelid problems such as lids turning outwards(ectropion) and lids turning inwards (entropion).
4) Eye allergies.
5) Preservatives in topical eye drops
6) Wind, smoke and dry air.
6) Vitamin A deficiency

Risk factors

1) Being older than 50 years. Tear production tends to decrease after the age of 50.
2) Lack of tears is more common in women, especially if they are experiencing hormonal changes due to pregnancy, using birth control pills and after menopause.
3) Eating a diet low in vitamin A and omega-3 fatty acids. Vitamin A-rich foods are carrots, liver, and broccoli.

Omega-3 fatty acids are found in fish, walnuts and vegetable oils.

4) Wearing contact lenses.

Prevention

If the problem of dry eyes arises, kindly look for the situations that might be causing it. Then, avoid those situations to prevent dry eyes. Following are the examples-

1) Air blowing directly in the eyes due to hair dryers, car heaters, air conditioners or table fans directed towards the eyes.
2) Winter season has dry air, causing dryness of skin and eyes. Add moisture to the indoor air using a humidifier.
3) Windy outdoor activities can cause dry eyes. Consider wearing sunglasses or other protective eyewear. Safety shields can be added to the tops and sides of the eyeglasses to block wind and dry air. Ask for shields where you buy eyeglasses.
4) The air at high altitudes, in desert areas and in aeroplanes can be extremely dry. When spending time in such an environment, it's helpful to frequently close the eyes for a few minutes at a time to minimise the evaporation.
5) Incorrect position of the computer screen-

   If the computer screen is above eye level, eyes are opened

wider to view the screen. Position the computer screen below the eye level so that wider opening of the eyes can be prevented.

6) Smoking and smoke-

Active or passive smoking can increase the symptoms of dry eyes.

Use artificial tears regularly if you have chronic dry eyes. Use them even if your eyes feel fine to keep them well-lubricated.

Treatment-

Occasional or mild dry eye symptoms require regular use of artificial tear eye drops prescribed by the Ophthalmologist, depending upon the type and severity of the dry eyes.

Some treatments focus on reversing or managing the factors or conditions causing dry eyes, while others concentrate on improving the quality of tears produced in the eyes or stopping the tears from quickly draining from the eyes.

F] <u>Allergic eye disease.</u>

Allergic eye disease or allergic conjunctivitis is caused by exposure to substances like pollen grains of flowers. The composition of the particles in the air changes with the change in the seasons. These particles include pollen grains, spores, dust particles and pollutants. They cause red, itchy and watery eyes.

Allergic conjunctivitis is very common. It is the body's reaction to substances it considers potentially harmful.

Types-

Allergic conjunctivitis is of two types-

1) Acute allergic conjunctivitis

   This is a short-term condition causing eyes to suddenly swell, itch, and burn when exposed to certain allergic substances.

2) Chronic allergic conjunctivitis

   This is a persistent type of allergic conjunctivitis which might occur around the year. It is a response to allergens like dust and animal dander.

   Common symptoms include burning, itching and sensitivity to light.

Causes of allergic conjunctivitis-

Allergic conjunctivitis occurs when a body perceives a threat and tries to defend itself.

It does this in the reaction to things that trigger the release of histamine.

Histamine is produced by the body to fight off foreign invaders.

Substances causing this allergic reaction are-

Household dander

Pollens from trees and grass

Spores

Animal dander

Chemical scents such as household detergents or perfume.

Some people may also experience allergic conjunctivitis in reaction to certain medications or solutions put in the eyes, such as contact lens solution or medicated eye drops.

People at risk are the ones who are usually more prone to allergies.

If such people live in a region with high pollen counts, they are more susceptible to allergic conjunctivitis.

Symptoms

1) Red, itchy, watery eyes
2) Burning sensation in the eyes
3) Grittiness in the eyes
4) Sensitivity to the light
5) Swollen eyelids
6) Puffy eyes in the morning

Treatment

Upon perceiving the symptoms, kindly consult your ophthalmologist.

Depending upon the severity, they can advise the following.

Care to be taken at home-

Avoid rubbing the eyes as it aggravates the symptoms.

Instil artificial tear drops to rinse the eyes.

Cold compress to relieve the inflammation and discomfort.

Wear sunglasses and had to offer some protection from the pollen grains.

Shower after coming in from outside if pollen is the trigger.

A thorough hand wash before touching the eyes, especially after handling pets or other sources of allergens.

Medications- The following medications are commonly used in allergic conjunctivitis, which should be strictly used after consulting an Ophthalmologist.

i) Antiallergic eyedrops reduce or block the histamine release.

ii) Anti-inflammatory eyedrops

iii) Eyedrops to shrink congested blood vessels.

Long term approach-

The treatment provides relief from the symptoms. Symptoms also disappear if exposure to allergens is avoided.

Recurring exposure to the allergens will likely trigger the same symptoms in the future.

Complications are rare in the allergic conjunctivitis. In the long term, some patients might experience damage to the cornea, and this may affect their vision.

Prevention-

The best prevention from allergic conjunctivitis is to avoid exposure to environmental triggers.

Depending upon the trigger, the following measures might help-

Use only scent-free soaps and detergents.

Install an air purifier in the home.

Vacuum and dust regularly.

Limit the carpets, soft toys, curtains and soft furnishings at home.

G] Vitamin A deficiency-

Vitamin A deficiency causes night blindness in children. It is worsened if it is combined with protein-energy malnutrition, causing severe corneal destruction.

Vitamin A deficiency always is associated with other nutritional deficiencies.

Vitamin A deficiency is of two types-

a) Due to a diet deficient in vitamin A.

b) Due to defects in the absorption and utilisation of vitamin A and other nutrients in diseases like- malabsorption syndrome, chronic liver diseases, chronic pancreatitis and severe infections.

Age group- Pre-school children are more vulnerable. Children between 2-3 years are mostly affected.

Gender- Males are more susceptible to vitamin A deficiency than females.

Socioeconomic status- There is a positive correlation between lower socioeconomic strata and vitamin A deficiency.

Physiological status- Pregnant and lactating women are more vulnerable. Consequently, lower vitamin A content in breast milk contributes to an increased risk of its deficiency in infants.

Diet – Rice-dependent communities suffer mostly from vitamin A deficiency.

Season- Vitamin A deficiency disorder, along with protein-energy malnutrition, occurs mostly in the summer season.

Breastfeeding- breastfeeding is highly protective against vitamin A deficiency. The composition of the weaning diet is also of great importance.

Cultural factors- Customs practised by the community are also of importance regarding dietary habits.

Infectious diseases- The important diseases predisposing the development of vitamin A deficiency are- diarrhoeal diseases, intestinal parasites, respiratory diseases like pneumonia, whooping cough, measles, and HIV/ AIDS.

Prevention of vitamin A deficiency-

In vulnerable children, an inexpensive and readily available vitamin A-rich diet should be given. Periodic administration of a large dose of vitamin A at an interval of 4-6 months to ensure adequate vitamin A storage in children. As vitamin A is a fat-soluble vitamin, it is stored in the fat cells of the body.

Sources of vitamin A-

1) Vegetable sources-

   Dark green leafy vegetables

   Spinach *(Remember Popeye?!!)*

   Carrot

   Tomato

   Pumpkin

2) Animal sources-

   liver

   meat

   cod-liver oil

   shark liver oil

   egg yolk

3) Fortified food items- vitamin A enriched commercially available food items.

H] Lazy eye, also known as Amblyopia-

Lazy eye or amblyopia is decreased vision in one eye, which usually starts developing in the early stage of life.

The age group when the lazy eye develops is from birth to seven years of age. It is one of the leading causes of decreased unilateral vision in children. Usually, the eye which is lazy, develops a squint.

We have two eyes, but the image of an object we normally see is one because there is a complex mechanism involved behind it. The eyes need to work in perfect synchrony to focus on the same object. One eye gives only a two-dimensional view. The presence of two eyes aids us in better depth perception and better analysis of the distance, which is also known as three-dimensional vision (3D). Most commonly, laziness goes undiagnosed for many years as the brain automatically focuses on the vision provided by the better eye for better visualisation and to avoid confusion. So many times, the lazy eye gets diagnosed only in the eye examination in the hospital.

The following are the symptoms of the lazy eye-

1) The eye movements are not coordinated.
2) The lazy eye has an inward or outward squint.
3) The child shuts one eye for better vision.
4) Decreased depth perception.

5) The child tilts head to one side for better vision.

6) Vision screening reveals lesser visual acuity in one eye compared to the other.

If the above symptoms are seen in the children, they should undergo an eye examination. For all children in the age group of 3 to 5 years, an eye examination is recommended.

The following are the causes of the lazy eye-

The development of the lazy eye happens due to poor development of the vision pathway between the eye and the brain. The weaker eye receives lesser visual inputs, while the better eye receives more visual inputs. So, the brain automatically focuses on the better eye and suppresses the weaker eye to avoid confusion resulting from the dissimilar images provided by the two eyes.

Any reason that causes the eye to squint or to have lesser vision can cause the lazy eye. The common causes are-

a) Difference between the vision of both the eyes-

   If only one eye has an undiagnosed higher spectacle number due to near-sightedness (myopia), far-sightedness (hypermetropia) or astigmatism, it results in a lazy eye.

   Diagnosis at an early stage and treatment with the correct spectacle number recovers the lazy eye.

b) Squint due to ocular muscle problems-

   The ocular muscle weakness interferes with the coordinated

movements of the eyes and causes one of the eyes to move inwards or outwards.

c) Obstruction in the conduction of vision from the eyes to the brain-

The most common cause of the obstruction is the cataract and corneal opacities in the paediatric age group. It should be diagnosed and treated at the earliest to avoid permanent vision loss.

The following are the risk factors for amblyopia-

a) Family history of lazy eye.

b) Premature birth

c) Developmental problems.

Treatment of the lazy eye includes the use of spectacles and contact lenses of the appropriate power and patching the better eye as suggested by the ophthalmologist.

CHAPTER 7

Eyes and occupational hazards

At the workplace, eye injuries are very common. There are many job-related injuries that require medical treatment.

Correct use of safety protocols can lessen the incidence and severity of eye injuries.

Entry of chemicals or foreign objects and scratches over the cornea are the common eye injuries that occur at work. The source of injuries is fluids entering the eyes, steam burns and ultraviolet or infrared radiation exposure.

In addition to that, healthcare workers, laboratory and janitorial staff and other workers may be at risk of acquiring infectious diseases from eye exposure. Some of the infectious diseases can be transmitted through the mucous layer of the eyes. This can occur due to direct contact with the splashes of blood, respiratory droplets generated during coughing or by touching the eyes with contaminated fingers or other objects.

The ocular injuries to the workers are due to the following reasons-

1) Due to not wearing proper eye protection
2) Due to wearing the wrong kind of protection for the given job.

It is revealed in the regular surveys that three out of five workers were not using eye protection during the time of the accident and have suffered eye injuries. These workers most often reported that they thought eye protection was not necessary during work.

The Occupational Safety and Health Administration (OSHA) requires workers to use eye and face protection whenever there is a reasonable probability of injury that could be prevented by such protective measures. Personal protective eyewear such as goggles, face shields, safety glasses or full-face respirators must be used when the possibility of an eye hazard exists. The necessary eye protection depends upon the type of hazard, the circumstances of exposure, other protective equipment used and individual vision needs.

Common professions requiring eye protection-

- Welders
- Miners
- Construction workers
- Carpentry
- Automobile repair
- Plumbing
- Welding
- Electrical work
- Drivers

- Doctors
- Computer professionals
- Farmers
- Water Divers
- Chemical laboratory technicians
- Pathology and microbiology laboratory technicians
- Teachers who use chalk and duster.

Potential eye hazards at work-

During the following potential eye hazards, workplace eye protection is required-

1) Projectile materials like dust, concrete, metal, wood and other particles.
2) Chemicals- fumes and splashes.
3) Radiation- visible light, ultraviolet radiation, heat or infrared radiation and lasers.
4) Blood-borne pathogens

   Hepatitis or HIV transmission through blood or body fluids.

Some working conditions include multiple eye hazards. Proper protective eyewear can take care of all the hazards.

How to protect the eyes from injury.

The following things can be done to protect the eyes from injury-

1) Knowing the potential hazards at the workplace.
2) Eliminate the hazards before starting the work by using machine guards, work screens or other engineering controls.
3) Use proper eye protection.
4) Keep the safety eyewear in good condition and replace it if it is damaged.

Selection of protective eyewear appropriate for the given task should be made based on the hazard assessment of each activity. Types of eye protection include-

a) <u>Non-prescription and prescription safety glasses-</u>

Although safety glasses may look like normal eyewear, they are designed to provide significantly more eye protection. The lenses and frames are much stronger than normal eyewear.

Safety glasses provide protection for the general working conditions where there may be dust, flying particles and chips. Side shields and wraparound-style safety glasses can provide additional side protection.

Safety lenses are available in plastic, polycarbonate and trivex materials. While all types of lenses must meet or exceed the minimum requirements for protecting the eyes, polycarbonate lenses provide the highest level of protection from impact.

b) Goggles-

Goggles provide protection from impact, dust, and chemical splashes. Like safety glasses, safety goggles are highly impact-resistant. In addition, they provide a secure shield around the eyes and protect against hazardous materials coming from any direction. Goggles can be worn over the prescription glasses and contact lenses.

c) Face shields and helmets-

Full-face shields protect workers exposed to chemicals, heat or blood-borne pathogens. Helmets are used for welding or working with molten materials. Face shields and helmets should not be the only protective eyewear. They need to be used in conjunction with the safety glasses or goggles so the eyes are protected when the shield is lifted.

d) Special protection-

Helmets or goggles with special filters to protect the eyes from optical radiation exposure should be used for welding or working with lasers.

Safety glasses must fit properly to provide adequate protection. Also, eye protection devices should be properly maintained. Scratched and dirty devices reduce vision, cause glare, and may contribute to accidents.

Combined with the machine guards, screened or divided workstations, and other engineering controls, using the correct protective eyewear can help maintain safety from any type of eye hazard.

Contact lenses usage in industrial jobs-

Contact lenses can't provide a significant amount of protection from eye hazards in the workplace. Contact lenses may actually increase worker productivity because they often provide improved vision in the workplace. Individuals who wear contact lenses have a wider field of vision than those with the glasses. They often have less visual distortion. In addition, wearing contact lenses can improve the fit and comfort of eye safety equipment such as goggles and full-face respirators. The workers must wear eye protection over contact lenses according to the requirements for all workers performing the same job.

What should be done in the case of an eye emergency?

Seek medical attention as soon as possible following the injury, particularly if the is blurring of vision, loss of vision or pain in the eyes. First aid steps should be taken until medical assistance is available.

First aid for the chemicals in the eyes-

1) Immediately rinse the eye with copious water. For that, pour water into the eye with a clean container.
2) Immediately remove the contact lenses if the person is wearing them before giving the eye wash.

3) Do not try to neutralize the chemical with other substances.

4) Do not bandage the eye.

First aid for the particles in the eye-

1) Do not rub the eyes

2) Try to let the tears wash the particles out or irrigate the eye with the artificial tear solution.

3) Try inverting the upper eyelid outwards and down over the lower eyelid to remove the particle.

If the particle does not wash out, seek medical help.

The metallic particles should not be tried to be removed at the workplace. They should be compulsorily treated by the Ophthalmologist. Do not delay the medical care in such cases.

First aid for the blows in the eyes-

Gently apply the cold compress without putting pressure on the eyes. Crushed ice in a plastic bag can be

Placed gently on the injured eye to reduce pain and swelling.

In case of severe pain or reduced vision, seek immediate medical care.

First aid for cuts and punctures to the eye or eyelid-

Do not wash your eyes

Do not attempt to remove an object that is stuck in the eye.

Cover the eye with a rigid shield like the bottom half of a paper cup.

Seek immediate medical care.

CHAPTER 8

Spectacles, Contact lenses and Refractive surgery

Teri pyaari pyaari surat ko kisi ki nazar na lage... Chashme-baddur!

Spectacles and contact lenses are an important aid for people with refractive error.

Spectacles are also an important beauty accessory to enhance the looks! Cosmetic contact lenses are also of importance in the beauty industry.

Let's learn more about them.

A] Importance of regular eye check-up-

The eyes are the most important sense organs of our body. They contribute to the maximum information of the world we live in. At the same time, they are also one of the most delicate organs of the human body. We need to take extra care of them, so regular eye checkups are very important.

The common belief among people about an eye examination is a vision checkup. But when you go to an Ophthalmologist, there is much more to an eye examination other than the vision checkup.

Depending on your Ophthalmologist and your medical history, a comprehensive eye examination consists of the following-

a) Vision checkup-

In an eye hospital, a vision checkup is done to see whether you have normal vision, near-sightedness or far-sightedness. Depending upon the examination, the prescription for spectacles is given.

Also, after the age of 40, near-vision spectacles are required by most of the population to see near objects clearly. That is also diagnosed during the regular eye checkup.

b) Slit lamp examination-

The slit lamp is a must equipment in the eye opd, which is an advanced microscope with built-in illumination. The minute structures of the eyeballs can be examined in an increased magnification to see the structures of the eyeball. The retina and optic nerve are also examined using this equipment.

c) Intra-ocular pressure recording-

The intraocular pressure of the patients is also recorded in the eye patients as a regular examination or in the suspected glaucoma patients. A rise in intraocular pressure is an important feature of glaucoma.

d) Retina examination-

The retina is examined in detail using a direct ophthalmoscope or indirect ophthalmoscope. It can also be done with the help of a slit lamp.

B] Importance of regular eye checkups in children-

School projects for the eye examination of children are imperative to diagnose the refractive errors in them. Many times, only one eye has a refractive error, and the other eye is normal. The brain captures and focuses on the image of a normal eye automatically, so the refractive error in the other eye never gets noticed by the kids or the parents, as the vision is normal when both eyes open.

Regular eye examinations also reveal the squint in the children. Squint treatment has a better result when it is diagnosed at an earlier stage.

Children who are already diagnosed with refractive error and have been using the spectacles should visit Ophthalmologist every 3-6 months, as advised. The children in the growing age group are expected to undergo changes in the refraction in a few months. Regular checkups ensure that they are using the correct refractive power (spectacle number).

Children using incorrect spectacles or not using the spectacles, in spite of having spectacles, are more prone to the increase in the spectacle number. They also tend to perform at a lower capacity in academics, as the majority of them cannot see the board or the projector clearly in class.

Many children are too shy to use the spectacles as they are teased by their peer group. Regular motivation should be given by the parents, family members and teachers to ensure that the child is using spectacles correctly and constantly.

Fun fact- There is also a regular number of kids who come to the OPD saying they are not able to see properly because they want to use the spectacles to look like a movie character or they want to use spectacles because their best friend has got spectacle!! Such false cases also need to be ruled out and counselled properly by the Ophthalmologist without hurting them or scolding them.

Myth buster-

There is a common misconception in society that the regular use of spectacles reduces their refractive power. This happens only in a fraction of patients with spectacles whose refractive power is less and of a specific type.

C] Importance of spectacle usage above the age of 40 years-

Above the age of 40, the power of the eyes to focus on the near and intermediate objects gradually reduces. This condition is called Presbyopia.

With the use of appropriate near-vision spectacles, this vision can be rehabilitated.

Types of the near vision spectacles-

1)Bifocal spectacles- These are the spectacles with different zones for the distant and near vision. The distant vision zone is upwards and the near vision zone is below.

These were the types of spectacles used before the invention of progressive spectacles a few years back.

The disadvantage of the bifocal spectacles is that they can focus only at a specific near distance. So, it is mandatory for the user of bifocal spectacles to hold the object of near-vision work at a fixed distance, irrespective of the type of work.

For example, the distance for the reading of the book is not equivalent to the distance used for cutting vegetables, though they both come under the category of near work.

Bifocal spectacles still served their purpose till the end of the 20th century, when the most common use of near vision spectacles in the form of bifocal spectacles was for reading books and newspapers.

The game changed with the advent of different screens, namely- cell phones, desktops, laptops, and tablets.

Then came the advanced version of near-vision spectacles known as Progressive spectacles.

2) Progressive spectacles-

These are the newer generation spectacles designed to focus on distant, near as well as intermediate distances.

These spectacles are a boon for computer users above 40 years, as the progressive spectacles focus on the intermediate distance where the computer screens are placed. Prior to the invention of progressive glasses, puter users above the age of 40 had to use a special unifocal spectacle to focus on the screen. But that spectacle couldn't be used on the distant as well as near vision. This caused difficulty in the day-to-day life of the middle-aged group of computer users as they had to carry one bifocal spectacle and one computer-use spectacle.

Progressive spectacles are very effective in daily life as the middle-aged computer user can simultaneously focus on the person addressing him from a distance (which is distant vision), on the laptop in front of him (which is intermediate vision) and the newspaper on his table (which is near vision).

D] Spectacle usage in screen users-

The spectacles are quintessential for screen users. The screen users' eyes are already tired due to long working hours at an intermediate distance. If they have a refractive error, even of mild grade, it causes straining if spectacles are not used. Spectacles help to focus on the pixels of the screen, which are clearer in the centre and blurred towards the periphery.

The spectacles with blue block glasses also help protect the retina from harmful blue rays.

Many screen users with minor refractive errors don't feel it is important to use spectacles for screen usage as they can manage their other activities without spectacles. This misconception causes them to suffer from eye strain. Eye strain typically increases towards the evening, causing a decrease in the employee's productivity.

Regular spectacle usage, even if it is of minor refractive error, helps them to cope with the long working hours in a better way.

E] Contact lenses usage and its care:

Contact lenses are commonly used for the correction of refractive errors as well as an accessory to enhance beauty!

Following are certain methods to keep contact lenses clean for the safety of your eyes.

a) Cleaning of the contact lenses-

The most used contact lenses are soft lenses. The disposable contact lenses do not require to be maintained.

1) Before handling the contact lenses, you should wash your hands thoroughly. If there is oil or lotion on the fingers, it can create a film on the contact lenses. This causes blurring of the vision as it interferes with the clarity and irritation in the eyes. After the hands are washed, they should be dried with a clean and lint-free napkin to avoid the entry of fibres in the eyes or over the contact lenses.

2) Contact lenses should be cleaned with the solution designated for its cleaning and not by tap water or filter water, as it increases the chances of infection.

3) When the make-up is supposed to be applied, lenses should be worn after the make-up is done, and the lenses should be removed before the makeup is cleansed.

4) Use of hair spray should be done before wearing contact lenses.

5) The nails of contact lens users should be clean, short and blunt to avoid tearing the contact lenses and injury to the eye while wearing the lenses.

E] Refractive Surgeries.

In simple term refractive surgeries are done to get rid of the spectacle number, usually done in the young adults.

The common refractive surgeries are LASIK, SMILE, PRK.

Among these, LASIK surgery is widely known so we will discuss LASIK as an example of the refractive surgeries.

LASIK stands for Laser assisted in situ keratomileuses. It is a widely known procedure for the correction of refractive error.

a) Pre-requisites for the LASIK surgery-

1) The age of the patient should be a minimum of 18 years complete, preferably more than 21 years, as in most of the patients, the refraction gets stabilised by then.

2) The thickness of the corneas should fulfil the criteria for LASIK. LASIK cannot be done in the thinner corneas.

3) The spectacle number should be stable for a one-year minimum. In unstable refraction, LASIK cannot be done.

4) The refractive error should be in the treatable range

of LASIK. Patients with extreme levels of myopia, hypermetropia and astigmatism are not good candidates for LASIK.

5) Patients should not have dry eye disease.

6) LASIK is contraindicated in patients with corneal diseases, cone-shaped cornea(keratoconus), corneal scars, cataracts, retinal disorders, advanced glaucoma, and uncontrolled diabetes.

7) Breastfeeding and pregnant ladies should not undergo LASIK due to vision changes that might happen due to hormonal changes.

b) To determine whether the person is a good candidate for LASIK, the following examination is done-

1) The latest refractive power is determined.

2) Corneal thickness is checked.

3) The retinal examination is done.

If all the above factors are normal, then the patient is scheduled for LASIK surgery.

c) Postoperative care includes-

Postoperative care should be done properly for the success of the surgery.

1) During the surgery, the upper part of the cornea is treated with lasers after creating a thin flap, and the flap is restored.

The flap heals itself.

During the healing process, rubbing of the eyes should be avoided, and the eyes should be kept protected with goggles.

2) The post-operative eyedrops should be instilled from time to time as advised by the Ophthalmologist for faster healing and care after the surgery.

3) Regular follow-ups are very important after the surgery for vision checkups to assess the health of the eyes and determine if any changes should be made in the postoperative care plan.

4) Avoid watching mobile and computer screens for a few days after the surgery.

5) While taking a bath, care should be taken to avoid the entry of water or soap inside the eyes.

6) Don’t drive until the Ophthalmologist suggests.

7) Don’t squeeze the eyelids forcefully.

CHAPTER 9

Eye donation

Any book or talk or knowledge about eye care is incomplete without the noble topic of eye donation.

Just close your eyes for five minutes and try to do your daily activities. It's so tough, right? Imagine the life of a blind person who has to struggle to live every day in the darkness when the fast-paced world around him or her is busy doing their own work.

Eye donation is a supreme act of donation as it allows someone to see this beautiful world and its amazing wonders when you are gone.

Eye donation done by one person gives sight to two blind people who have corneal blindness.

Eye donation is a voluntary act done by a person for the benefit of society, from which patients of corneal blindness are benefitted.

a) <u>When and by whom the eye donation can be done-</u>

Eye donation is accepted from a person after his death who has filled out the form and given consent for the same. The person should let his or her family know about his or her decision so that the family can inform the eye bank after his or her death. Ideally, the eye donation procedure should be done within 6 hours of the death.

After the death of any person who has not filled out the eye donation form, the close relatives can also choose to donate the eyes of their deceased relative.

In the procedure for the eye donation, the entire eyeball is not removed; only the corneas are removed, and the lids are properly stitched to close them, so there is no disfigurement to the face of the person who has passed away. The procedure only takes 15-20 minutes.

There is a waiting list for the recipients in the eye bank, according to which the corneal transplantation surgery is done. The eyes are never sold. Eye donation is never refused by the eye bank.

There is no age limit for the eye donation. A person of any gender, religion, or socioeconomic status can donate the eyes. A person who has undergone cataract surgery or any other eye surgery can donate the eyes with the prior intimation. The identity of both the donor and receiver is kept anonymous. The service of eye donation is provided free of cost by the government and the NGOs.

b) Who cannot donate eyes-

A person suffering from-

AIDS, hepatitis, encephalitis, rabies, septicemia, leukaemia and retinoblastoma.

c) Steps of the eye donation process to be done by the kins of the deceased person-

A call should be made to the nearest eye bank as early as possible.

The eyes of the deceased should be closed and covered with moist cotton.

The overhead fan should be switched off to prevent the corneas from drying.

Any lubricating eye drops should be put in from time to time to keep the corneas clear and moist.

Antibiotic drops should be instilled to avoid any infection.

The head of the deceased person should be kept on a pillow to avoid bleeding during the procedure of eye donation.

Eye donation is a noble act by which one person can bring light to the lives of two different people and can drive off the darkness in their lives forever.

To increase awareness about eye donation and to make people all over the world know the importance of eye donation, 10th June is celebrated as International Eye Donation Day. National eye donation fortnight is observed in India in the last week of August and the first week of September. The first eye bank in India was started in 1945 at the Madras Eye Infirmary, now known as the Regional Institute of Ophthalmology, Chennai. It was set up by Dr. R.E.S Muthiah, who also performed the first corneal transplant in 1948. He is known as the Father of eye donation in India.

According to a recent survey by the Eye Bank Association of India (EBAI), India has 1.1 million people with corneal blindness. These people will benefit from the corneal transplants.

The celebrities who have pledged their eyes are-

Superstar Rajinikanth

Amitabh Bachchan

Aishwarya Rai Bachchan

Priyanka Chopra

Salman Khan

Rani Mukerji

Aamir Khan

Alia Bhatt

CHAPTER 10

Interesting facts and myths about the eyes

INTERESTING FACTS ABOUT HUMAN EYES-

1) The natural guards of our eyes-

The eyes are one of the most delicate organs; therefore, in evolution, many protective mechanisms for the eyes have been evolved. Our eye sockets are inside the skull, thereby half of the eye is protected from behind by the bones of the skull.

The eyebrows protect the eyes from the sweat entering the eyes from the forehead. Also, the eyebrows shield the eyes from the sunlight falling in the eyes directly above the head. The hair of the eyebrow is touch-sensitive, which initiates the protective reflex of closure of eyelids when they come in contact with any foreign body.

Our eyelashes act like guards by protecting the eyes from the dust like the filters. They are also touch-sensitive, so when any external material comes in the vicinity of the eyes, they send the message to the brain to close the eyelids. The entire length of the eyelashes shed in a lifetime is 98 feet. Each eyelash has a lifespan of almost 5 months.

The eyelids are like curtains of the eyes, which close on any slightest hint of the possibility of harm to the eyes.

Even if all these protective armours are provided to us by evolution, we are not well equipped with protection against modern hazards like industrial traumas and intense artificial light. For the protection against these, we need to use special eyewear in these environments where the possibility of trauma to the eyes is higher.

2) There is a blind spot in our vision-

Yes, that's true! Even if we feel that we can see everything, we all are blind in a tiny specific zone of our peripheral vision. That zone is created in our visual field due to the area where the retina is pierced by the optic nerve along the blood vessels of the eye.

We hardly ever experience blind spots because of binocularity. The blind spot of one eye is covered by the vision from the other eye, so there occurs the overlapping of the vision and the blind spot of both eyes is covered by each other. Just like two best friends who are always there for each other, to cover each other's lacunae and magnify each other's strengths! The blind spot coverage is one of the important advantages of having two eyes!

3) Red-eye in the photos is due to the blood vessels in the eye-

We all hate when we are the ones with the red eyes in a group photo, impersonating like some Halloween ghost!

There is also a special feature in cell phones to correct the red eyes! There is so much use of technology to hide or correct natural phenomena!

The red-eye effect occurs when the light of a camera flash is another bright light reflected back at the camera. The light which is reflected illuminates the blood vessels of the eyes, which produces the red colour we see in the photos.

So next time you have a photo with the red reflex, just relax, it's totally natural!

4) Sunburn in the eyes-

Just like the skin gets sunburned, the eyes are also susceptible to sunburn by intense sunlight, especially at higher altitudes. The signs and symptoms include pain, watering, redness and irritation in the eyes. In severe cases, the upper layer of the cornea might just peel off, causing extreme pain.

So, in higher altitudes, the use of protective sunglasses with ultraviolet A and ultraviolet B protection is very important. Also, they provide a great style statement for the perfect snaps on the picturesque snow-clad mountains!

5) Getting a near vision spectacles-

The common misnomer in society is that getting near vision spectacles is equivalent to old age ringing your doorbell!

After the age of 40, the natural crystalline lenses in our eyes lose their power to focus on objects nearby. This intensifies after the age of 50 years. This condition can be rectified by the use of near-vision spectacles.

6) **How good carrots are for the eyes?**

We all grow up with a very common belief that carrots are superfoods for the eyes and can cause wonders for vision.

Even though it's true that carrots are a rich source of vitamin A, they are not the only rich source. Vitamin A is required for the maintenance of normal vision and the development of the eyes. The other rich sources of vitamin A are spinach, avocado, fish oils, and other green leafy vegetables.

Carrots will definitely boost the vitamin A in the body but will not improve the existing vision or make it flawless.

7) **Computer vision syndrome-**

Computer vision syndrome is a group of symptoms due to prolonged exposure to digital screens. This includes straining of the eyes, pricking, burning, and redness in the eyes. This can be avoided by a simple rule of 20-20-20.

When there is a prolonged time to be spent on the screens, intermittently look at a distance of 20 feet every 20 minutes for 20 seconds. This will provide great relief from computer vision syndrome and will increase the quality of life of screen users during working hours.

8) **Many vision impairment problems can be cured-**

According to the World Health Organisation (WHO), many eye diseases around the world can be treated or prevented. The WHO highlights a number of successful public-private partnerships that have improved eye health across the globe. There has been a substantial decrease in eye infections, trauma, and visual rehabilitation due to the awareness generated over a period of time.

9) Our blink rate is almost 25000 per day-

We blink on an average 25000 times per day. Each blink lasts for just two-tenths of a second but is equivalent to 45 minutes per day. Blinking removes the dirt from the eyes and also lubricates the eyes. It is also postulated that the brain resets and refocuses its attention when blinking happens.

10) The size of the eyeball determines the type of refractive error-

If a person has a shorter eyeball length, he develops hypermetropia or farsightedness. In hypermetropia, the rays of light focus behind the retina instead of being focused on the retina.

A person with a longer eyeball length develops myopia or near sightedness. In this condition, the rays of light focus in front of the retina instead of focusing on the retina.

In both cases, the resultant image formed is blurred. The use of appropriate spectacles focuses the image exactly on the retina and helps the person to see better.

11) Iris scans are the best for the security purpose-

The iris scans are better than the fingerprints in the biometric systems. Like the fingerprints, the iris scans are also unique for each individual. Our irises have 256 unique characters compared to the fingerprints, which have only 40. That's why iris scans are more secure.

12) Eye colour does not affect the vision-

The quality and quantity of the vision is not dependent on the eye colour. Blue and green eyes are more sensitive to light compared to brown eyes. The brown eyes have more melanin, which absorbs the light better.

13) Human eyes can detect 10 million different colours-

We, as humans, can distinguish between 10 million different colours. The colours visible to the human eyes are within the light spectrum, and they are in the combinations of red, green and blue. It is not just the wavelength of the light but also our perception in relation to the background colours, lighting, familiarity and surroundings.

14) Eyes are filled with a jelly-like substance-

The jelly inside our eyes is called the vitreous humour. It is maximum made of the water and is a clear jelly to aid the normal vision. Vitreous homor occupies the hollow space between the lens and the retina, provides shape to the eyeball and supports the retina.

15) The eyes see things upside down-

When the light rays pass through the cornea, the rays are bent in such a way that when the image reaches the retina, it's inverted. But when it reaches the brain, it again rectifies it so that we can see the world erect!

FUN FACTS ABOUT ANIMAL EYES

1) An owl can see a moving mouse more than 150 feet away.
2) A worm has no eyes at all.
3) Guinea pigs are born with their eyes open.
4) Shark corneas are similar to the human eyes.
5) Scorpions can have as many as 12 eyes, but the box of jellyfish has 24!
6) Camels have three eyelids, this is to protect their eyes from sand blowing in the desert.
7) Most hamsters only blink one eye at a time.
8) Owls are the only bird species which can see the blue colour.
9) Goats have rectangular pupils to give them a wide field of vision.
10) A scallop has around 100 eyes around the edge of its shell to detect the predators.
11) Snakes have two sets of eyes- one set used to see and the other to detect heat and movement. They also don't have eyelids, just a thin membrane covering the eyes.
12) Owls cannot move their eyeballs- which has led to the distinctive way they turn their heads almost all the way around.

13) The four-eyed fish can see both above and below the water at the same time.

14) A dragonfly has 30,000 lenses in its eyes, assisting them with motion detection and making them very difficult for predators to kill.

15) Dolphins sleep with one eye open.

16) The largest eye on the earth belongs to the Colossal Squid, it measures around 27cm across.

17) Geckos can see colours around 350 times better than the humans, even in the dim lighting.

18) The eyes of the chameleon are independent of each other, allowing it to look in two different directions at once.

19) A camel's eyelashes can measure up to 10 cm long to protect its eyelashes from sand and debris in the desert.

20) An ostrich’s eye is bigger than its brain.

21) Dogs can't distinguish between red and green.

22) Polar bears have a third eyelid, which helps filter the UV light.

23) Human eyes are not the most highly evolved. The mantis shrimp has four times as many colour receptors as the human eye, and some can see ultraviolet light.

24) Pigeons can see millions of different hues and have better colour vision than most animals on Earth.

25) Cats' eyes have almost 285 degrees of sight in three dimensions, which is an ideal peripheral vision for hunting.

26) Although colour- blind the cuttlefish can perceive light polarization, which enhances their perception of contrast.

27) A moth's eyes are covered with a water-repellent, anti-reflective coating.

28) An ant only has two eyes, but each eye contains many smaller eyes, giving it a compound eye.

29) Eagles have 1 million light-sensitive cells per square millimetre of the retina- humans only have 2,00,000.

30) A honeybee's eye is made of thousands of small lenses. A drone may have up to 8600, and the queen bee can have 3000-4000 lenses.

31) The night vision of tigers is 6 times better than that of humans.

32) The eyes of the horses and the zebras point sideways, giving them tremendous peripheral vision, to the point of almost being able to see behind them.

MYTHS AND MYTH BUSTERS

There are very commonly found myths in society which have become popular. Here are some common myths and their bursters.

1) *Myth-If the eyes are crossed willingly while having fun, they will remain in the same manner!*

   Fact-

   Very commonly, children, while playing, cross their eyes to make funny faces, or clowns or comedians do it to add drama to their act. Our eye muscles allow us to move our eyes in any direction, like up and down or left and right. If the eyes are crossed willingly, there is no permanent damage caused to them. It's very much natural to move them according to our will.

   In diseases related to the nerves of the eyes, in uncorrected vision or in eye muscle trauma, the eyes are crossed or squinted. They need treatment from an Ophthalmologist.

2) *Myth-Looking directly at the sun will sharpen your eyesight.*

   Fact-

   Locking the eyes with the sun or looking directly into the eyes of the sun is considered a heroic feat! In reality, looking at the sun directly without using proper eye protection might damage the retina. Of course, we can admire and appreciate the beauty of the inspiring sunrise and poetic sunsets when the sun's rays are milder and softer. But even looking at the morning or evening sun cannot improve the sight.

Solar retinopathy is a very common reason for vision loss seen due to watching the solar eclipse without using proper protective glasses. Only ISO-certified goggles should be used to watch the solar eclipse. Routine sunglasses or homemade filters are not recommended.

3) *Myth-Carrots are a superfood to improve eyesight.*

Fact-

Carrots are rich in Vitamin A, which is essential to maintain a healthy vision. There are other foods that are rich in Vitamin A, like spinach, dairy products, and fish. While eating foods rich in vitamin A can help us maintain healthy vision, it won't improve the vision or prevent the use of spectacles. Vitamin A-rich food should be combined with good fats to help better absorption.

4) *Myth-Eyesight can be improved with the eye exercises.*

Fact-

Eye exercises prescribed by ophthalmologists are for convergence insufficiency, a condition resulting from the inability of the eyes to focus on near objects, causing strain. These exercises improve the muscle tone of the eyes, helping them focus better while reading. However, they don't improve the eyesight or preserve it. Having a healthy vision is dependent upon multiple factors. None of those factors are significantly altered by the eye exercises.

5) *Myth-Babies are born with their eyes fully grown.*

Fact-

When babies are born, almost two-thirds of the growth is completed. But they continue to grow from birth till puberty. That is why children who have spectacles should be examined every six months, as the changes in refraction are expected when they grow up.

6) *Myth- Colour-blind people can see only in black and white.*

Fact-

Colour blindness is a genetic disorder in which there is an insufficiency to distinguish between colours. Most commonly, there is difficulty in recognising the green and red shades. Most colour-blind people are partially colour-blind. The most severe form of colour blindness, where everything is seen in shades of grey, is very rare. Boys are more affected than girls.

Colour-blind people are born with a partial or complete lack of specific cones in the retina, which are responsible for distinguishing the red, green and blue colours. Very uncommonly, colour vision problems can occur later in life due to diseases of the retina, trauma, and toxic effects of drugs.

7) *Myth- Reading in the dim light will decrease the vision.*

Fact-

There is no effect on the vision if one reads in the dim light. However, it is advised to read in an adequately lit environment for better visibility and to avoid straining the eyes. The retina of our eyes is equipped with special types of cells called rods to assist us in night vision. But for the clarity, contrast sensitivity and detailing of the objects, light is required. In the light, the cells of the retina, known as cones, are functional.

8) *Myth-Eyes are transplanted completely.*

Fact-

Only the cornea, which is the transparent part of the anterior eyeball, is transplanted. The entire eyeball cannot be transplanted as the eye is a complex organ connected to the brain with the optic nerve.

Once the connection with the optic nerve is broken, it cannot be re-established.

As only the cornea can be transplanted, blindness occurring due to eye diseases related to the cornea can only be cured by the transplant.

9) *Myth-Cataracts should be removed only when they are completely mature or ripened.*

Fact-

Cataract surgery after the complete maturity of the cataract used to be done almost thirty to forty years back when the surgical methods didn’t have the fortification of the technology.

In today's world, this concept is obsolete.

Thanks to the newer and refined surgical techniques of cataract surgery, the cataract can be removed as soon as it hampers functional vision and interferes with the routine of the patient.

Due to the invention of superior-quality intraocular lenses, visual restoration is of supreme importance after cataract surgery.

A few decades back, when intraocular lenses were not used, thick spectacle usage was imperative after the cataract surgery. But today, cataract surgery is incomplete without the implantation of the intraocular lens.

10) *Myth-Using spectacles will make you dependent upon them.*

Fact-

The use of spectacles will not worsen our eyesight or increase our dependency on them. On the contrary, they aid in better vision and help in our day-to-day lives.

Distant vision spectacles in people with refractive errors are required for better learning and safety while driving or working.

Near-vision spectacles are a must after the age of 40 for most people to help focus on near-vision objects. Today, the majority of the work is on computers and mobiles. So, the use of near-vision spectacles is very important.

The capacity of the human eyes to focus on near objects decreases gradually from the age of 40 till the age of 55.

So, the near vision spectacle number increases as the age advances beyond 40 years. It is misinterpreted by many that the near vision spectacles have increased their dependency on the spectacles whereas it's just an age-related change.

11) *Myth-If the upper or lower eyelid of the right eye twitches, it's a good sign, and you will be getting money soon. If the upper or lower lid of the left eye twitches, it's a bad omen.*

Fact-

This is a myth and has multiple variations depending upon the region and the person who says this!

In reality, the twitching of the eyelids is due to physical and mental stress or due to decreased levels of potassium in the body.

As the muscles in the eyelids are tiny compared to the other muscles in the body, they get fatigued sooner. Having a combination of a healthy diet, better exercise, and meditation can help you avoid twitching of the lids.

12) *Myth-Looking at greenery improves the eyesight.*

Fact-

Looking at the greenery does not have any added advantage to looking at red or blue things! Yes, it does give a cooler sensation, but it does not improve the existing eyesight. Looking at a distance relaxes our eye muscles. So, it's not necessary to look at a tree; you can look at any distant object instead. Looking at a distance of 20 feet for 20 seconds every 20 minutes is advised by Ophthalmologists to relieve the strain caused by focusing continuously on the computer or mobile screen.

13) Myth-Having a vision of 6/6 or 20/20 means your eyes are healthy and perfect.

Fact-

The vision of 6/6 or 20/20 means that only the central vision is perfect. There are other aspects to the vision, such as peripheral vision, night vision, and colour vision. These may be affected by diseases like colour blindness, diabetic retinopathy, and glaucoma. It takes years for these diseases to deteriorate vision, so a regular ophthalmological check-up will have a better prognosis for these diseases.

14) *Myth-Cataract occurs only in the elderly.*

Fact-

Even though old age is the biggest contributor to the cataract, other age groups are not immune to it.

Cataracts might develop as a result of developmental disorders in children. Cataract also develops after an eye trauma. In diabetics and prolonged steroid users, it can develop at a younger age. Certain professions involving heat and radiation can also contribute to the development of cataracts.

15) *Myth-Reading for a longer duration can decrease the eyesight.*

Fact-

Our eyes are special sensory organs designed to see, so they won't wear out when they are used more. Just like the nose doesn't get tired of smelling and ears don't get tired of hearing, eyes also never lose their power of seeing by seeing more. Intermittent breaks from reading are recommended to relax them and relieve the tiredness.

CHAPTER 11

"Oh! I See" Moments.

As an Ophthalmologist, I get many moments of realisation in my daily OPD. Here are a few of them I would like to share. Some are bone-tickling and hilarious, while others provoke me to think deeply. (Names of the patients are changed.)

1) A 10-year-old boy was brought to my OPD by his parents with the complaint of itching in both his eyes. I examined him and gave him an eyedrop to instil for a week and told him to visit again after one week. When he came back after a week, his parents complained to me about him. They said he had not been instilling the eyedrops for a few days.

   I asked the boy why he was not using the eyedrop. He said, " Madam, I am really relieved a lot with the medication, but when I close my eyes after instilling the eyedrops, I fall asleep! So to avoid falling asleep, I don't use the eyedrops."

   I was deeply puzzled. How is that possible?

   I thoughtfully asked him, "For how many minutes do you close your eyes after putting the eyedrop?"

Upon that, he gave such a hilarious answer that I couldn't control my laughter.

He said," For the better effectivity of the eyedrop, I close my eyes for half an hour instead of 2 minutes!! I just don't realise when I fall asleep!!"

Me-*"Oh, I see!! "*

When the eyedrop is put in the eye, only one minute of closure of the eyelids is enough. Also, the common question asked by the patients is how many drops from the bottle of eyedrops are to be instilled in a single eye at a time. The answer is only one eyedrop. Many times, patients feel that the eye does not get enough medication with a single drop. So, they put two to three drops from the bottle. These extra eyedrops, anyway, roll out of the eye as the space available in the eyelids for carrying the medication is only for one drop. So, a single drop is enough. Also, putting more drops from the eyedrop bottle also leads to economic loss as the eyedrop bottle will become empty sooner, and the patient will be required to purchase another one to complete the specific days of medication.

If two or more types of eyedrops are prescribed, then a single drop from each is enough, with a gap of at least 5 minutes in between so that each individual eyedrop gets time to act and get absorbed. If two or more types of eyedrops are put immediately after the other, all the eyedrops will roll out of the eye, and their efficacy will be decreased as the time for acting inside the eye is lesser.

2) One of the common incidents in an Ophthalmologist's OPD is parents coming to me complaining that their kids watch mobile phones a lot. On asking the kids in detail, I came across many variations of answers.

Scenario-

Me- "Hello Sandy! Tell me why you want to spend so much time on your mobile phone."

Sandy- "Madam, I just want to pass my time after I am done with my studies."

Me- "So why don't you read the books?"

Sandy- "In my home, everyone spends their time on the mobile screen, and no one reads a book in our home, so why should I?"

Me- *"Oh! I see..."*

In today's world, cell phones have become a source of massive information and communication. From watching the newspaper to watching the daily entertainment, everyone uses their mobiles.

So, the habit of regularly reading newspapers, comics,

storybooks, and magazines in printed form is becoming less and less.

The advantage of reading in the printed form, for example, a storybook, is that our brain uses its imagination to set the background of the story as well as to put colours to the characters and the personalities. When we read, we apply our full concentration and attention. Our memory also becomes strong, and we tend to remember better whatever we read in the tangible form.

Whereas if we see the same story on a screen, our brain is fed with readymade food. So, literally, there is no food for the thoughts. The thinking and self-visualisation power of our brain is not put to use. The use of cell phones in moderation in today's world is acceptable. Kids can see their cell phones for a maximum of 30 minutes a day. But outdoor playing activities and reading books are very crucial for their mental and physical growth.

Also, our kids will not follow what we preach to them, but they will follow what they observe us doing on a regular basis. So, if we want our kids to read more books, we have to read more! We must become the example that we want our kids to follow.

3) A middle-aged man, Mr. Joshi, came to the OPD to get his old parents examined.

Scenario- After I examined both his parents,

Mr Joshi- "Madam, I want to say something."

Me- "Yes, please go ahead."

Mr Joshi- "Madam, I want to complain to you about my parents that they watch cell phones a lot! Please tell them not to use mobiles!"

Me (trying very hard not to laugh!!)- "Respected Aunty and Uncle, may I know the reason for your excessive mobile usage?"

Joshi Aunty and Uncle- "Dear Madam, we are both over 65 years old. In the good old days, we didn't have this technology. So, we are making the most of what we have missed!"

Me- *"Oh! I see..."*

The middle-aged population of today's era have a common problem with their kids as well as their parents, which is unhindered screen usage! These days, the older population have increased screen usage. It's been a real boon to them in terms of reconnecting again with their long-lost childhood and college friends, as well as the use of technology at their fingertips and various entertainment options available on mobile phones. But the problem always lies in the excess of anything. Over usage of social media, watching online videos, and watching episode after episode on streaming platforms are becoming harmful in many ways.

The cognitive abilities of the brain are depleting faster due to excessive screen time. The memory loss is setting in faster. As far as the eyes are concerned, dryness is very common in the elderly due to continuous watching of the screen. The decreased blink rate during screen usage increases the dryness of the eyes, which is already present in most of the geriatric population due to old age-related changes.

The use of technology and social connectivity is fine only when done in moderation and until it does not physically harm the elderly.

4) A young IT professional, Ms Sneha, came with the complaint of eye-straining and a pricking sensation in the eyes.

Ms Sneha- "Good morning, Madam; my eyes are getting tired soon, and I feel a gritty sensation in my eyes."

Me- "How many hours of screen time do you have?"

Ms Sneha- "Work-related screen time is almost 8 to 9 hours, and then cell phone use for social media and entertainment is 2 hours. So, a maximum usage of 11 hours is the maximum."

Me (after examining her)- "That's a very huge screen time.

This itself is the culprit. I will prescribe you an eyedrop, which you are supposed to put four times a day."

Ms Sneha- "But I don't have time to put the eyedops. I am busy working all the time."

Me- "*Oh! I see!* Dear Sneha, if you have time in between tea and water breaks, lunch breaks, and also ample mini breaks for browsing social media, you will definitely find time for the instillation of eyedrops!"

Many IT professionals or other professionals requiring more screen time have the screen time induced dry eye, for which we Ophthalmologists prescribe eyedrops. They have a common query of not having time to instil the eyedrops. It takes only half a minute to instil eyedrop and close the eyes for a minute. That time can be easily spared by anyone in between work as we already take breaks in between and are not glued to our chairs and tables continuously for 10-12 hours. Also, instilling eyedrops for screen users with dry eyes is essential in between their work as the screens are the main culprit for their symptoms.

Eyedrops provide great relief to screen users, and they also increase work productivity by relieving the eyes of the symptoms of tiredness and pricking sensations while working.

5) Mrs. Meena, a mother of a 2-year-old girl, came to the

OPD to get her daughter's eyes examined.

Mrs Meena- “Doctor, my daughter just doesn’t leave the cell phone. She wants to watch the cartoon videos all the time.”

Me- “But she is just 3 years old, why do you give her the cell phone?”

Mrs Meena- “It just started with giving her the cell phone while eating, and now she wants it all the time.”

Me- *“Oh! I see.”*

This is a very common scenario these days with kids of very early age, as young as 7-8 months old, having their meals, watching nursery rhymes, and playing on their cell phones. This trend is very dangerous in toddlers and kids as the screens are habit-forming. The use of screens is addictive. It activates the same centres in the brain as the addiction-forming substances do. That's why the kids have a typical behavioural pattern of getting irritated and even getting agitated when someone removes the cell phone from their hands.

Also, the use of cell phones interferes with the development of the brain and its learning abilities.

The minds of small kids are very innocent; they get addicted to the screen more easily than adults.

The kids who regularly watch the screen have higher

chances of getting spectacles and a faster increase in the refractive power of already existing spectacles.

The initial years of age are prime for the development of eyes. More playing with the toys to increase their cognitive abilities and outdoor activities are recommended for the development of the knowledge about the outer world, also for the physical development.

It's a common scene all over, that kids are refusing to go to play outdoors as they find it more enchanting to play on the screens.

Screens also lead to a decrease in the attention span of the brain, leading to poor learning skills in school.

A stitch in time saves nine. So, parents should refrain from handing over their mobiles to babies and kids at a young age to avoid eye problems and behavioural problems as they grow.

6) A retired uncle, Mr. Gupta, complained of a burning sensation in the eyes and tiredness of the eyes after waking up.

Mr. Gupta- "Doctor, I am experiencing fatigue and burning in my eyes after waking up. Also, I have a restless sleep. I don't fall asleep easily, and even when I sleep, it is disturbed."

Me – "What is your schedule these days?"

Mr. Gupta- "I have no specific schedule as I am retired now. I spend most of my time watching entertainment videos and catching up with my friends on social media.

Me- Do you watch the mobile screen before sleeping and immediately after waking up?"

Mr. Gupta- "Yes, I watch entertainment programs on my mobile at night to pass my time as I don't fall asleep easily. In the morning, I have to wish good morning to so many of my friends and relatives on social media."

Me- *"Oh! I See!"*

Ocular problems related to screen usage are so many.

The dryness of eyes due to unhindered digital screen usage causes the eyes to get tired and have a burning sensation, as we tend to blink less while using screens.

The blue light from the screen is very notorious. Regular exposure to blue light causes damage to the cells of the retina and, over a period of time, causes macular degeneration, decreasing vision.

The blue light from the screen also disrupts the sleep pattern by decreasing the production of melatonin, which is a brain chemical required for the normal sleep pattern and circadian rhythm. People with decreased sleep watch screens to pass their time, leading to more disruptive sleep, hence setting in the negative vicious cycle.

Ideally, two hours before sleeping and two hours after waking up, the screens should not be used to help the normal circadian rhythm.

7) Mr Sunil was brought to the OPD by his friends with a complaint of iron particle entry in the left eye during welding. He had severe pain, redness and watering in the eye.

Me- "Hello, Mr. Sunil; when did the iron particle enter your eye?"

Mr Sunil- "It entered yesterday."

Me- "Then why didn't you come to the OPD yesterday itself?"

Mr Sunil- "I tried to remove it myself yesterday and thought my pain would be relieved, so I waited for one day. But my pain and watering has increased."

Me- *"Oh! I see!"*

The cornea is a very delicate and sensitive structure in the eyes. Entry of iron particles in the eye during welding happens if the proper eye protective goggles and shield are not used.

If the iron particles enter the eye, they should be removed by the Ophthalmologist with the help of an OPD microscope known as a slit lamp. If the removal of the iron particle is not done on the same day, a rust ring forms behind the particle in the deeper layer of the cornea. Moreover, the iron particle is sharp and can cause further trauma to the eyes if the patient rubs the eyes. An attempt to remove the iron particle by the patient or other people can cause irreversible damage to the eyes, causing permanent loss of vision.

Any particle in the eye needs to be removed by an expert Ophthalmologist to avoid trauma and infection to the eye.

8) Mrs. Deshmukh, a 55 year old lady came to the OPD with the complaint of watering in both the eyes.

Me- “Hello, Deshmukh Aunty. Since when do you have watering in the eyes?”

Mrs. Deshmukh- “It's been there for 15 days. I am instilling this eyedrop prescribed for my husband one year back.”

Me- “But why didn’t you discard the eyedrop bottle?”

Mrs Deshmukh- “Because the expiry date printed on the eyedrop bottle has not arrived yet.”

Me- *“Oh! I see!”*

The eyedrops, once opened, should be used for a maximum of 4 to 6 weeks. The expiry date is given so that they should be opened before the date and not be used till the date of expiry.

Once the eyedrop bottle is opened, the preservative in it works only for a few weeks, and then it starts depleting. Also, the pharmacological actions of the eyedrops decrease once the preservative becomes ineffective. If kept for many months after opening, the eyedrop might cause untoward effects in the eyes. This might result in a serious problem or aggravate the existing problem for which the patient instilled the old eyedrop.

The patient should discard the eyedrop after the therapeutic dose is instilled for a number of days, according to the Ophthalmologist's advice.

Any eyedrop previously used by a family member or friend should not be used to self-treat as it may worsen the eye problem. All the eyedrop bottles look almost the same, but the eyedrops inside them have varied properties. Certain eyedrops used for treating a specific disease can be an absolute contraindication in the other type of eye disease. So using the eyedrops for self-medication kept at home casually and unmonitored, is a strict no-no.

9) Mrs Usha came with the complaint of a decrease in her near vision for a few months. She was accompanied by her college-going son Atul.

Mrs Usha- "Madam, I cannot focus on the near objects

when I am stitching or doing kitchen work."

Me- "Ok. Please tell me, what is your age?"

Mrs Usha- "I am 30 years old!"

Me (trying not to look shocked)- "What?" (As of we now know, near vision decreases gradually, mostly after the age of 40 years)

And then, out of nowhere her son spoke…

Atul- "But mom, I am 20 years old!!!! Don't bring me along if you want to hide your age!"

Me – *"Oh! I see!"*

It is a very common and funny incidence in the OPD of an Ophthalmologist that few patients are forever 30 to 35 years old. They might have passed the 40 years of their chronological age long back, but still, they refrain from admitting their true age!

The near vision spectacle power increases as the age increases after 40 years and is different for the different age groups. So, if the patients tell us the correct age, we Ophthalmologists are in a better position to prescribe them the correct near vision spectacle number!

Honesty is the best policy!

"THANK YOU, I LOVE YOU AND KEEP SMILING UNTILL WE MEET NEXT TIME!!"

References

1) Parsons' Diseases of the Eye

   Editors Ramanjit Sihota and Radhika Tandon

2) Anatomy and Physiology of the Eye

   K. Khurana and Indu Khurana

3) History of Ophthalmology

   American Academy of Ophthalmology

   Article by Peng Yong Sim.

4) 32 facts about animal eyes

   Discovery eye foundation

   Aug 5, 2014

5) Ophthalmic contributions of Raja Serfoji II (1798-1832)

   Indian Journal Of Ophthalmology

   Jyotirmay Biswas, Vasanthi Badrinath and Sengamedu S Badrinath.

6) Eye diagram- The college of optometrists. Parts of the eye- Eye Anatomy.